THE CLINICAL MANAGEMENT OF MUSCLE DISEASE

A Practical Manual of Diagnosis and Treatment

THE CLINICAL MANAGEMENT OF MUSCLE DISEASE

A Practical Manual of Diagnosis and Treatment

IRWIN M. SIEGEL, MD* FACS FICS

**Senior Attending Orthopaedic Surgeon and Chairman, Department of Orthopaedic Surgery, Strauss Surgical Group Assoc., L. A. Weiss Memorial Hospital, Chicago, Illinois*

Clinical Associate Professor, Department of Orthopaedic Surgery, The Abraham Lincoln School of Medicine, University of Illinois, Chicago, Illinois

Director, Muscle Disease Clinic, University of Illinois, The Medical Center, Chicago, Illinois

Director, Muscle Disease Clinic, L. A. Weiss Memorial Hospital, Chicago, Illinois

Medical Consultant, Muscular Dystrophy Association, Inc.

WILLIAM HEINEMANN MEDICAL BOOKS LTD
LONDON

First published 1977

ISBN 0 433 30275 5

Text set in 11/12 pt Photon Times printed by photolithography,
and bound in Great Britain at the Pitman Press, Bath.

This Book Is For

PORCIA

Who Should Know Why

Acknowledgements

It is a pleasure to acknowledge my gratitude to Mrs Alice Thanner and Mrs Jacqueline Jukish for their secretarial assistance in the preparation of this manuscript. Indebtedness is also due the Women's League for Crippled Children, Louis A. Weiss Memorial Hospital, Chicago, Illinois and the Muscular Dystrophy Association, Inc. for their financial support. I also wish to thank Mrs Rose Sirks, Secretary, Muscle Disease Clinic, University of Illinois, as well as Mrs Irja Hetzel, RN, Mrs Thelma Eager, RN, and Mrs Daria Harris who so ably staff the Muscle Disease Clinic at Louis A. Weiss Memorial Hospital, Chicago, Illinois. Finally, my sincere appreciation to my father, Allen Siegel, and to Louis Goldstein for the illustrations and the Department of Photography at the University of Illinois Medical Center for their photographic expertise.

Contents

Preface

Since poliomyelitis has ceased to be an epidemic problem in the United States, other crippling musculoskeletal diseases have gained increasing attention from pediatricians, internists, orthopaedic surgeons and physiatrists. Muscle diseases, particularly the muscular dystrophies, though not a major problem numerically, have increasingly engaged the attention and efforts of these and related specialties. Currently, there are approximately 10,000 children with Duchenne muscular dystrophy living in the United States. The incidence of risk has been estimated as approximately 270 cases for each one million live male births. The occurrence of limb girdle dystrophy is approximately 65 cases per 1,000,000 births (male or female), and that of facioscapulohumeral dystrophy, 4 cases per 1,000,000 of either sex.

This monograph is not a comprehensive treatise on the diagnosis and treatment of muscle disease, nor does it present differential diagnosis and therapy in depth. Encyclopedic texts on this subject are available elsewhere. Rather it was written in response to the need for a compendium of the general problems of muscle diseases, offering a concise diagnostic method and outline of therapy. Although every facet of treatment (physical, social, psychiatric, etc.) is covered, emphasis is directed toward physiatric and orthopaedic therapeutic techniques. No effort is made to summarize even briefly the vast ongoing body of research literature, and, except when necessary for a better understanding of clinical problems, theory is not discussed. Instead, the practical aspects of diagnosis and care are stressed.

Many children are misdiagnosed early and see three or more physicians before a correct diagnosis is made. This needlessly delays vital genetic counselling and sometimes important therapy. It is hoped that this small volume will amend this situation by providing a ready desk or bedside reference, enabling the practicing physician to outline and organize the sometimes confusing nomenclature and voluminous literature on muscle disease, reach a diagnostic category with facility, and apply treatment appropriately.

Unfortunately, the cause of these diseases has not as yet been discovered, and until a cure is found, all therapy must be palliative. Nonetheless, supportive and symptomatic aids are available, and through early diagnosis and proper therapy, comfort, functional capacity, and even life expectancy can be significantly increased.

Finally, I hope this brief text will dispel some common errors of belief concerning Duchenne muscular dystrophy—such 'myopathic myths' include the misconception that it is exclusively a disease of boys and the fallacy that nothing can be done for the disease.

It has been aptly stated that: 'we cannot as yet prevent a child from having muscular dystrophy, but we should never allow muscular dystrophy to have the child.' Seeing that muscular dystrophy never 'has a child' presents a continuing challenge to all practitioners called upon to care for these patients.

CHAPTER 1

Clinical Diagnosis

INTRODUCTION

The muscular dystrophies are genetically determined, primary, degenerative, myopathic diseases.* Abiotrophy, with subsequent atrophy and weakness of striated musculature (particularly that of the proximal 'limb-girdles'), is the common feature of the muscular dystrophies.

These conditions are characterized by a progressive clinical course, lacking signs of central or peripheral involvement of the nervous

* Recent laboratory research has suggested neurotrophic and angiopathic influences in the evolution of some muscular dystrophies.

Chart 1. A Working Classification of the Common Diseases of Muscle

*Type**	*Age of Onset*	*Sex*	*Symptoms*	*Course*	*Miscellaneous*
Childhood dystrophy Severe-(Duchenne) Benign-(Becker) Later onset, slower progression	1 to 4 years	Male, primarily	Clumsiness, toe-walking, lordosis, Gower's sign, pseudo-hypertrophy	Increasing weakness with contracture, wheelchair by age 8 to 10, death in late teens	Mental retardation – 25% abnormal EKG – 50%
Limb-girdle dystrophy	Any; commonly 2nd to 3rd decade	Equal	Extensor weakness, shoulders and hips	Slow progress with late disability	Occasional pseudohypertrophy
Fascioscapulohumeral dystrophy (Landouzy-Dejerine)	2nd to 4th decade†	Equal	Paucity of facial expression, variable speech defect, difficulty in abducting arms, scapular winging, Bell's sign	Progressive weakness, very late disability	Variable life expectancy; little tendency to develop contractures
Dystrophia myotonica	Adult life†	Equal	Myotonia, lugubrious facies, severe fatigability, drop-foot gait	Slowly progressive weakness, temporal baldness, cataracts, gonadal atrophy, sterility, impotence, hypothyroidism, diabetes, acromegaly, hyperostosis cranii	Mildly progressive social and mental retardation

* Approximately one-third of all cases of muscular dystrophy occur sporadically. Other, less common, types include the ophthalmoplegic form, distal myopathy, central core disease, arthrogryposis, McArdle's syndrome and nemaline (rod) myopathy. Two distinct types of dystrophy in one family have never been reported.

† Can present in childhood.

(Adapted from Coodley, E. L. (Ed.) (1970), *Diagnostic Enzymology*. Philadelphia, Pennsylvania: Lea & Febinger, Chap. 9, p. 262.)

system, and without spontaneous improvement. A working classification of the most common dystrophies is presented in Chart 1.

The differential diagnosis of the muscular dystrophies includes secondary diseases of muscle, particularly polymyositis, as well as a variety of neuropathies. The most important of these are listed in Chart 2.

DIAGNOSTIC PROCEDURES

The diagnosis of muscular dystrophy is made on the basis of:

1. Genetic background.
2. Clinical history.
3. Physical examination.
4. Elevation of muscle enzymes.
5. Electromyographic studies.
6. Muscle biopsy.

Chart 3 with accompanying illustrations summarizes genetic determination of the most common types of muscular dystrophy.

Clinical History

Except in the case of the congential myopathies, the childhood forms of muscular dystrophy have a normal birth and developmental history. These patients are usually asymptomatic until three to five years of age, at which time a significant enough mass of muscle (upwards of 33%) is lost to impair function. Often enough such children are first seen by practitioners unalert to or unaware of the possibility of muscle disease. They are presented as a problem of gait which is frequently treated only symptomatically (e.g. corrective shoes, exercise) and the basic diagnosis overlooked.

In general, the muscles first formed in the embryo are first involved in the dystrophic process. Axial and proximal muscles are weakened before their distal counterparts, the sternal head of pectoralis and lower trapezius before the remainder of these muscles. Extensor muscles are involved prior to their flexor analogues (Fig. 1).

The very first muscles to show clinical weakness are the extensor stabilizers of the shoulder girdle. However, because hip extensors play such an important role in maintaining pelvic-femoral stability, functional loss in these muscles with concomitant hip flexion contracture is

Chart 2. A Differential Diagnosis of Muscle Disease

Disease	*Features*
Polymyositis	See Special Section to Follow
Progressive Spinal muscular atrophy	Neurological disease(s) in which there is failure of development or progressive degeneration of the lower motor neuron cell body, with resultant degeneration of the peripheral motor nerve fibers, neurogenic atrophy, and paresis of the muscles innervated
Amyotonia congenita syndrome	An array of conditions characterized by muscular weakness, hypotonia, and variable degrees of hypermobility of joints, appearing at or shortly after birth
Benign congenital hypotonia 'Floppy baby syndrome'	Symptomatic hypotonia having a myopathic EMG pattern, which recovers partially or completely
Peroneal muscular atrophy (Charcot-Marie-Tooth disease)	Progressive muscular atrophy with onset from 1 to 50 years of age, characterized by equinovarus foot deformity
Acute anterior poliomyelitis	Typical clinical history of acute febrile disease, with scattered muscular involvement and non-progression
Flaccid cerebral palsy	Absence of familial history with occasional ataxia, mild spasticity, and other signs of CSP
Amyotrophic lateral sclerosis	Combination of upper and lower motor neuron signs and symptoms with intact sensation
Friedreich's ataxia	Rare familial degeneration of spinal cord and cerebellum of unknown etiology, characterized by unsteady gait, foot deformity, nystagmus, and kyphoscoliosis
Myasthenia gravis	Disease of myoneural junction with onset between 10 and 70 years of age. Ptosis common. Response to cholinergic drugs
Myotonia congenita (Thomsen's disease)	Hereditary condition characterized by delayed relaxation of muscles

Chart 2 (*Continued*)

Disease	*Features*
Metabolic disease accompanied by muscle weakness	Glycogen storage disease, thyrotoxic myopathy, menopausal muscular dystrophy, cerebral lipoidosis, steroid myopathy, diabetes
Kugelberg-Welander syndrome (Heredo-familial proximal spinal muscular atrophy)	Lower motor neuron disorder with weakness, wasting and loss of appropriate reflexes, particularly affecting the quadriceps, and (when the arms are involved initially) the triceps and biceps
Miscellaneous diseases associated with myopathy	Polyneuritis, collagen-vascular disorders (LE, RA, polyarteritis nodosa)

often noted first. Clumsiness, waddling gait, frequent falling, difficulty ascending stairs and rising from the seated position are usual complaints.

The history in the benign form of juvenile dystrophy (Becker's type) or in the adult dystrophies is essentially the same, but symptoms are of later onset and lesser severity.

Anamnesis in all cases should include birth and developmental history with particular attention paid to neonatal and natal 'at risk' factors. Parents are questioned to determine whether or not motor and

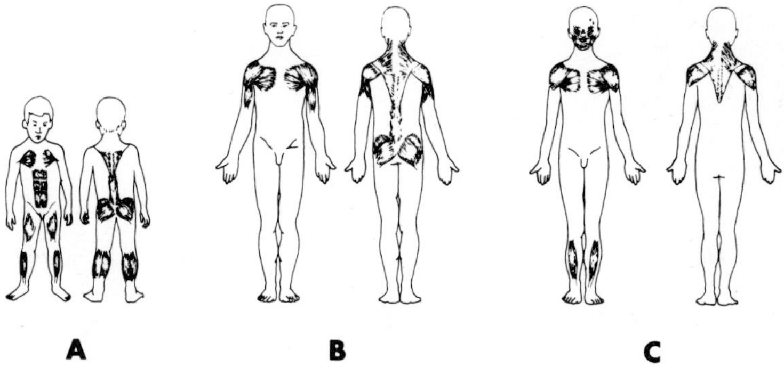

Fig. 1. Early distribution of muscle weakness in the three major forms of muscular dystrophy: (a) Duchenne dystrophy; (b) Limb girdle dystrophy; (c) Facioscapulohumeral dystrophy.

Chart 3A. Patterns of Genetic Determination for the most Common Types of Muscular Dystrophy

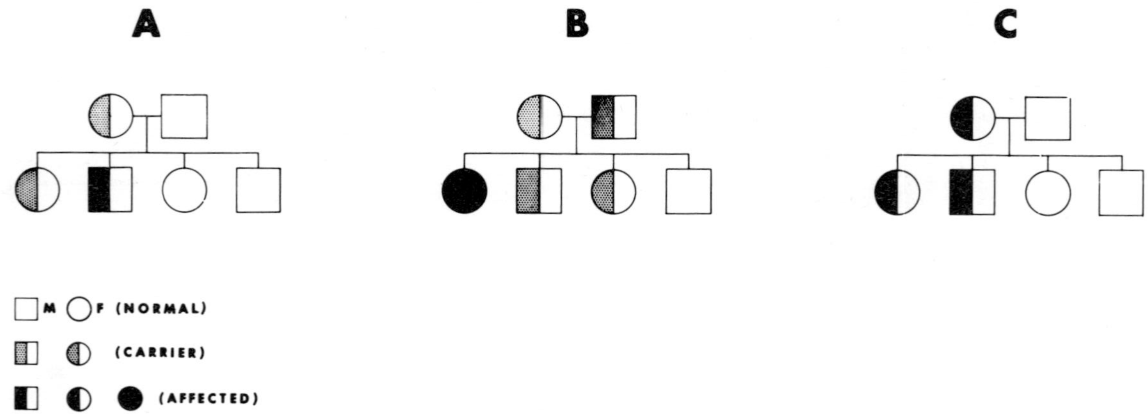

a.* X-linked heredity (classic Duchenne dystrophy), carried only by females and transmitted only to males. 50% risk of each male child having the disease and 50% risk of each female being born a carrier.

b. Autosomal recessive heredity (limb girdle Dystrophy). Both parents carry the defective gene. 25% risk (regardless of sex) of transmitting the disease, and 50% risk (again regardless of sex) of transmitting carrier state.

c. Autosomal dominant heredity (facioscapulohumeral dystrophy). Either parent has the disease (there is no carrier state). 50% risk for any child (regardless of sex) inheriting the disease.

* Were a male with X-linked dystrophic to procreate, none of his sons could have the disease, and all of his daughters would be carriers, unless of course his mate were a carrier, in which case each son would stand a 50% risk of inheriting the disease.

Chart 3B

Type	*Genetic pattern*	*Affected risk*	*Carrier risk*	*Miscellaneous*
Duchenne	Sex-Linked Recessive	Each Male 50%	Each Female 50%	One-third or more of all cases due to sporadic mutation
Limb girdle	Autosomal Recessive	Each Child 25%	Each Child 50%	Affected rise 100% if both parents exhibit clinical disease
Facioscapulohumeral	Autosomal Dominant	Each Child 50%	0	Fully penetrant trait
*Dystrophia myotonica**	Autosomal Dominant	Each Child 50%	0	Variable expressivity 'Formes Fruste' occur

* If the mother has the disease, it usually presents in an affected child at birth. If the father has the disease, it usually presents in an affected child in adolescence or young adulthood.

social milestones were met on time. Three fundamental areas of development, namely motor, language and adaptive social behavior should be historically assessed. A detailed familial history of similar or related disease, including close questioning regarding extrinsic causes of muscle weakness such as trauma, organic and inorganic toxins, drug intake, infections, or other such agents should be carefully pursued.

Inquiry is directed toward the occurrence of the childhood exanthems and conditions known to cause secondary muscle disease (e.g. diabetes). A careful nutritional and metabolic history must be taken. Present complaints and status should be assessed historically and intellectual state and personality determined. Figure 2 presents a check list for a complete muscle disease work up (history, physical exam., etc.).

Physical Examination

Duchenne Dystrophy

Examination of a young Duchenne dystrophic reveals symmetrical weakness with atrophy of the muscles of the pelvis and abdomen as well as the quadriceps. Unbalanced hip flexion contracture causes an increase in lumbar lordosis, and contracture of the tensor fascia latae leads to a wide based waddling gait. Heel cord tightness which early on causes flat feet, because the child cannot dorsiflex at the ankles and rockers the foot at the mid tarsal joints in an attempt to keep it plantigrade, later results in equinus steppage (Fig. 3).

Such patients tire easily and are unable to jump from the standing position. Other early signs include:

1. Weak neck flexion.
2. Difficulty in walking on the heels.
3. Awkwardness in sitting up.
4. Limited passive ankle dorsiflexion.
5. Some depression of deep tendon reflexes, except those of the Achilles tendons.
6. ‘Floppiness’ about the shoulder girdle leading to ‘slipping through’ when the child is lifted from the armpits.

Because of quadriceps weakness the patient cannot rise from the floor, except by climbing up his own legs in a manoeuvre known as the Gower's sign (tripoding) (Fig. 4). Although occurring in any patient with a similar distribution of muscle weakness, this sign is usually present in the child with Duchenne dystrophy.

Most weakened muscles are atrophic except the calves, where early hypertrophy and later pseudohypertrophy may be seen. This is occasionally present in the deltoids, triceps, and lateral vastei. Neck extensors and hamstring muscles are spared. Facial and extraocular musculature are intact. However, masseter hypertrophy as well as macroglossia severe enough to interfere with speech may occur. Cranial nerves are normal. Sensation is not affected. Tongue fasciculations are not seen nor is myokymia on muscle percussion, minipolymyoclonus,* or neostigmine induced muscle fasciculation (all usually evident in neuropathic disease). Reflexes are never brisk in weakened muscles and extensor plantar responses are never seen.

Involved muscles have a doughy consistency on palpation. Nonspecific changes may occur in the subcutaneous fat and the skin frequently shows a vascular flush (erythema ab igne).

As weakness progresses the deep tendon reflexes are lost. Those on the dominant side and in the ankles remain longest. Progression of weakness is relentless, and its rate appears to be inversely proportional to the age of onset of the disease. Weakness is accelerated by prolonged immobilization.

Limb-Girdle Dystrophy

Limb-girdle dystrophy occurs from late in the first through the fourth decade of life. Musculature of the shoulder and hip girdles is affected (Fig. 5). Onset is insidious and less rapidly progressive than in Duchenne type dystrophy. Patients occasionally complain of pain following activity which is related to excessive demand placed on involved musculature.

Prognosis is better in most patients who manifest shoulder weakness first. Pseudohypertrophy is unusual. Contractures are of late occurrence. The brachioradialis muscle is usually spared. Extensor digitorum brevis may be hypertrophied. Selective congenital absence of a single muscle can occur. Although the disease progresses slowly, most patients are incapacitated within several decades after onset.

Facioscapulohumeral Dystrophy (Landouzy-Dejerine Disease)

FSH muscular dystrophy makes its appearance at any time through the fourth decade of life. Facial weakness gradually results in the 'myopathic facies' characterized by inability to fully close the eyes

* A fine muscular tremor, usually noted in the outstretched hand, seen in neuropathy secondary to asychronous firing of reinervated muscle fibres.

MUSCLE DISEASE WORK-UP LIST

Name ______ Age ______ Occupation ______

Weight: Maximum weight with date ______ Average weight ______
Present weight ______ Weight loss or gain with duration ______

Birth and Developmental History:

a) Movement in utero ______
b) Length of Labor ______ Complications ______ Birth weight ______
c) At risk factors (Rh., etc.) ______
d) Convulsions ______ Jaundice ______ O_2 lack at birth ______

Motor Milestones:
Sitting ______ Standing ______ Walking ______

Symptoms:
Stairs ______ Run ______ Rise ______ Falling ______ Jump ______
Clumsiness ______ Rising from floor ______ Other ______
Shoulder, arm, and hand function ______
Description of gait (at onset of illness) ______

Family History:
Father ______ Mother ______ Brothers and Sisters ______
Cousins ______ Other relations with possible m.d. ______

Past Medical History:
First symptom noted (age) ______ saw M.D. ______
Original diagnosis ______
Prescriptions (medication, bracing, P.T.) ______
______
Progression ______
Other significant illnesses ______

Other development:
Intellectual ______ Personality ______

Cranial Nerve and Thoracic Involvement:
Facial musculature ______ Dysphagia ______ Dysarthria ______
Breathing ______ Frequency of respiratory infections ______

Development of Deformities:
Lower extremities ______ Upper extremities ______ Spine ______
______

Cardiorespiratory:
Palpitation ______ Dyspnea ______ Chest pain ______ Cyanosis ______
Dependent edema ______ Orthopnea ______ Cough ______

Gastrointestinal:
Eating habits ______ Appetite ______ Vomiting ______
Nausea ______ Pain or distress ______
Bowel habits and control ______

Neurologic:
Paresthesias ______ Pain ______
Muscle cramps ______ Trophic changes ______

Fig. 2a. Muscle disease work-up check list, part 1.

General Examination:

B.P.______ Pulse______ Respiration______ Temp.______
Nutrition and General Appearance______
Head______ Neck______ Skin______ Heart______
Lungs______ Chest______ Abdomen______
Spine______ Extremities______
Weakness and wasting______ Contractures______
Facial and extra-ocular musculature______
Neck musculature______ EENT______
Neurologic findings: Cranial nerves______ Sensory______
Reflexes______
Babinski______ Hoffman______ Bell's sign______
Fasciculations______ Myotonia______
Pseudohypertrophy______ Obesity______
Cataracts______ Baldness______ Fever______ Malaise______
Arthralgia______ Rash______ Tenderness______
Performance:
Run______ Jump______ Rise______ Gait______
Other______
Miscellaneous______

Laboratory Work-Up:

Enzymes______ Biopsy______
EMG______ EKG______
Other______
Physical Therapy______ Occupational Therapy______
X-Rays______

Social work-up______
Psychologist______ Dietician______
Other medical consultations______

Summary of Significant Findings:

______

Impression:

______

Plan for further work-up and treatment:

______

Fig. 2b. Muscle disease work-up check list, part 2.

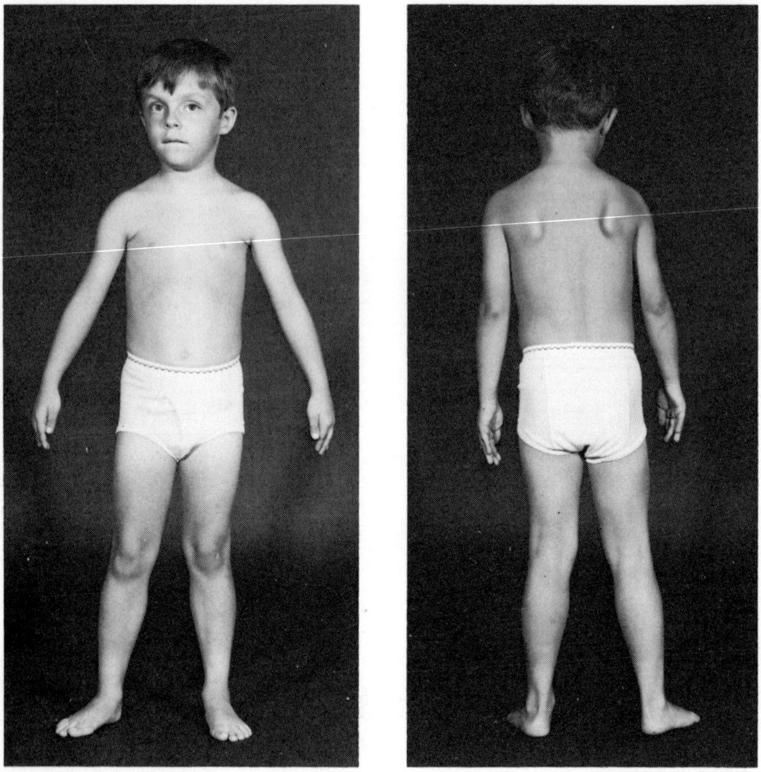

Fig. 3. Frontal and posterior views of young Duchenne dystrophic.

(Bell's sign), difficulty in pursing the lips (patients cannot whistle), 'tapir' mouth (lip eversion and protrusion), a transverse smile and inability to wrinkle the forehead or puff the cheeks (Fig. 6).

These facial signs are accompanied by weakness and atrophy of the shoulder girdle (deltoid is usually spared). At first unilateral shoulder weakness may be present. Weak finger extension may be an early sign and weak wrist extension can lead to the 'praying mantis' position of unopposed wrist flexion typical of the late disease. However, the forearms and hands are initially preserved and this results in so-called 'popeye arms' where muscles above the elbow are atrophied and those below appear larger because they are normal. Pelvic girdle musculature as well as tibialis anticus are also involved. Back extensors, tensor fascia and quadriceps are often exempt from the disease. Weakness is usually

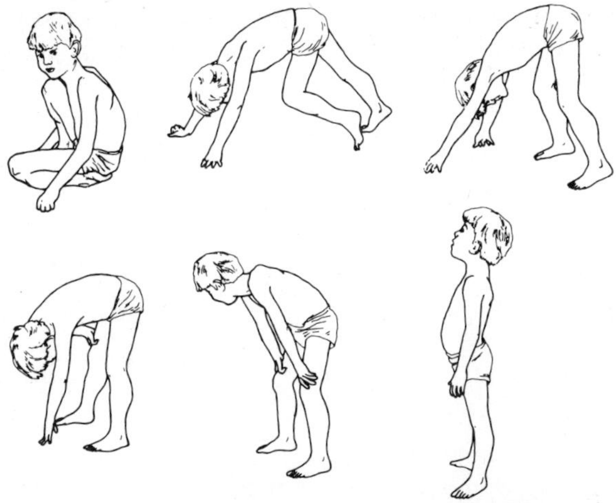

Fig. 4. Diagrammatic illustration of Gower's sign.

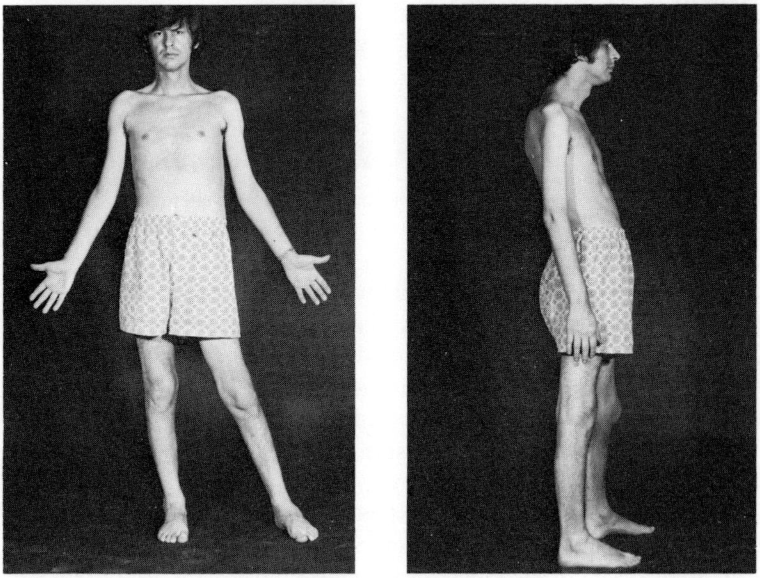

Fig. 5. Frontal and lateral views of patient with limb girdle dystrophy.

asymmetrical in distribution and degree. There is wide variability of clinical involvement both from family to family and from one patient to another within a given pedigree.

When it occurs in very early childhood, FSH dystrophy runs a rapidly disabling course. However, with usual adolescent or adult onset, progress is insidious and compatible with a normal life expectancy. Mentation is not affected.

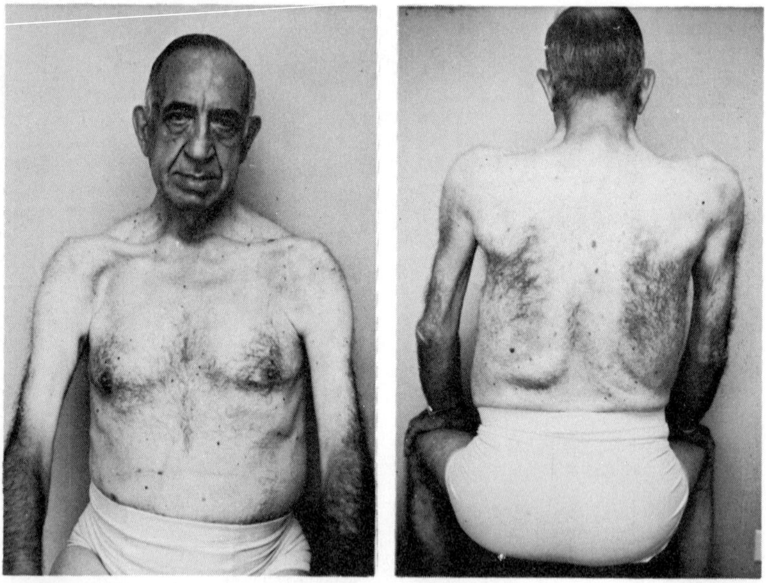

Fig. 6. Frontal and posterior views of patient with facioscapulohumeral dystrophy.

Dystrophia Myotonica

Most myopathies (distal myopathy excluded) are proximal (at least early in their onset) in distribution whereas most neuropathies are distal (Kugelberg-Welander Disease excluded). Dystrophia myotonica is an exception to this general rule. In this condition somatic musculature below the knee and elbow are affected in combination with a condition of myotonia (the inability of muscle to relax after contraction) noted particularly in the hand (slowness in release of grip), the tongue (dimpling on percussion) and the thenar eminence (myotonic contracture on percussion) (Fig. 7). Spasm of the globe elevators can also be seen after forced eyelid closure with sudden lid release. Myotonia persists even after nerve section, block or curarization. It is increased by cold or fatique but tends to lessen and sometimes disappear in the later stages of the disease because greater muscular weakness precludes severe myotonia.

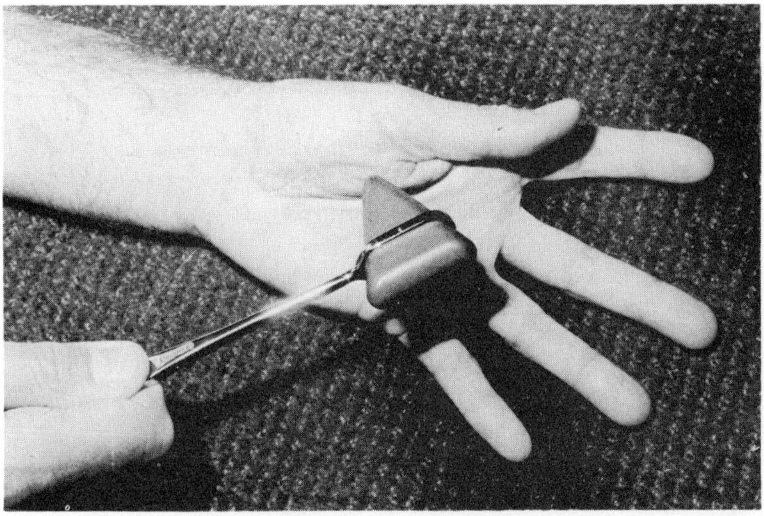

Fig. 7. Thenar myotonia.

The anterior strap muscles of the neck (particularly sternocleidomastoid) are weakened leading to 'swan neck'. The typical facies of dystrophia myotonica is diagnostic, consisting of a thin, haggard, expressionless face, transverse smile, inverted triangle ('shark') mouth, hollow temples and cheeks, ptosis and temporal baldness (Fig. 8). Dystrophy of the tibialis anticus is most disabling as it produces equinus. Foot drop causes the patient to stumble, myotonic spasm occurs and he falls. However, it is the weakness (dystrophia) and not the myotonia which troubles these patients the most.

Additionally, the syndrome includes:

1. Stellate cataracts.
2. A variety of skull abnormalities including enlargement of the paranasal sinuses, hyperostosis cranii, decrease in sella tursica size, prognathism and hyperostosis frontalis interna.
3. Progressive cerebral ventricular dilatation.
4. Gonadal atrophy (impotence in males, chronic abortion in females).

5. Impaired carbohydrate tolerance (diabetic glucose tolerance curve).
6. Low urinary creatinine excretion.
7. EKG abnormalities.
8. Decreased maximal breathing capacity (leading to nightmares) secondary to alveolar hypoventilation.
9. Dysarthria (secondary to tongue myotonia).
10. Neuronal Heterotopias.
11. Nasal speech (secondary to pharyngeal muscle weakness).
12. Dysphagia (because of pharyngeal myotonia).
13. Serum gamma globulin abnormality.
14. Low BMR.
15. Paranoid personality changes with a fall off of higher intellectual functions leading slowly but progressively to intellectual and social deterioration.

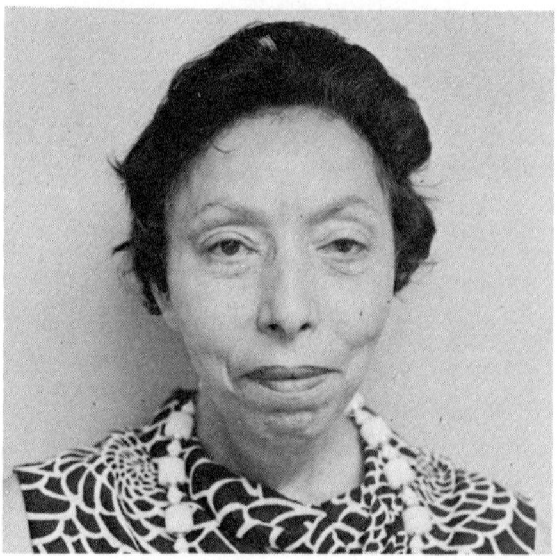

Fig. 8. Myotonic facies.

In dystrophia myotonica the apparently normal siblings of affected individuals tend on an average to die at a younger age than they should and (because of variable expressivity of this disease) correlation regarding severity between affected members of the same family is very low.

Myotonia congenita (see notes in Differential Diagnosis) as well as paramyotonia (syndrome of congenital myotonia with episodic weakness affecting all voluntary musculature and activated only by exposure to cold) should be considered in the differential diagnosis of this disease.

Although muscular weakness tends to be the major cause of disability in dystrophia myotonica when myotonia is troublesome a variety of drugs are available for relief. These include:

1. Quinine (dosage grains 5 t.i.d.).
2. Procaine amide (dosage 0.5 g to 1.0 g q.i.d.).
3. Prednisolone (dosage 10 mg b.i.d. to t.i.d.).

Diphenylhydantoin and even ethyl alcohol can decrease myotonia. However, no single case of a myotonic alcoholic has yet been reported. Physical therapy and bracing may be necessary and this treatment will be covered in the section on Therapy.

Other Less Common Forms of Myopathy

1. Distal Myopathy: Intrinsic musculature of hands and feet is weakened.

2. Occular Myopathy: Weakness of extraocular muscles, usually evident as ptosis or opthalmoplegia, often associated with dysphagia secondary to weakness of pharynx and esophagus.

3. Congenital Myopathies: A group of primary diseases of muscles which may be symptomatic at birth, presenting with weakness and hypotonia. Some do not appear until later in childhood. A positive family history is often elicited. The congenital dystrophies usually have a dysmorphic appearance (kyphoscoliosis, pigeon chest, pes cavus, high arched palate and an unusually long face). Diagnosis is made by special histological techniques which may include electron-microscopy.

This group of diseases includes central core disease, nemelene myopathy, mitochondrial disease, myotubular myopathy and congenital muscular dystrophy. Progression in myotubular and mitochondrial myopathy is very slow and characterized by progressive fatigability and weakness. Nemelene myopathy and central core disease are non-progresssive but motor development is marked by the slow acquisition of motor skills. In the severe form of congenital muscular dystrophy either death occurs in early infancy or profound residual weakness remains.

4. Myotonia Congenita: A familial disease characterized by delayed relaxation of voluntary muscle contraction, unaccompanied by weakness. This myotonia is aggravated by emotional stress and cold. The disease is nonprogressive and responsive to drug therapy (procaine amide or diphenylhydantoin). The myotonia tends to improve with age, being compatible with normal survival.

5. Arthrogryposis: This is a clinical observation and not a specific diagnosis. There are two types, neuropathic and myopathic. The condition is characterized by muscle weakness and joint contractures.

6. Miscellaneous: A variety of metabolic abnormalities including glycogenosis or glycogen storage diseases in which the excessive accumulation of glycogen resulting from the deficiency of a specific enzyme causes muscle weakness. Also a group of disorders characterized by attacks of paralysis with flaccidity which tend to remit and relapse known as periodic paralysis are recognized. Different types have been described depending on whether the serum potassium is low, normal or raised during an attack. These plus a variety of non-episodic endocrine, drug induced, collagen-vascular, neoplastic, infectious and granulomatous, nutritional, traumatic and vascular disorders, as well as a variety of ill-understood clinical syndromes (H^2O syndrome-hypotonia, hypomentia and obesity, stiff man syndrome, etc.) complete the differential diagnosis of muscle diseases causing weakness and atrophy.

Polymyositis

The diagnosis of polymyositis (one of the above noted collagen-vascular syndromes) is of more than academic interest, as this disease is responsive to steroid therapy whereas there is no known cure for the muscular dystrophies.

Polymyositis is a rare, non-suppurative, inflammatory disease of unknown etiology (although presumed to belong to the group of autoimmune conditions) and protean manifestations.

Approximately 50% of all cases of polymyositis are linked either with a collagen or connective tissue disorder or with a malignant tumour. Such malignant disease is usually found in a dermatomyositic male over 40 years of age. The tumour is most often a carcinoma (bronchogenic or prostatic in males, uterine, ovarian or mammary in females). Neoplasm is seldom found in the child with polymyositis.

The remaining 50% of these cases develop as primary myopathies or present as dermatomyositis. Angiopathic findings (e.g. Raynaud's phenomena) are present in those cases associated with collagen disorders, and rash with dermatomyositis. However, dermatomyositis may present with eyelid edema only. One must rule out myositities associated with other systemic diseases, such as viral, parasitic, etc. Thus, polymyositis is a member of those collagen-vascular disorders which include dermatomyositis, lupus ertythematosus, polyarteritis, rheumatoid arthritis and periarteritis nodosa.

In contrast with classical Duchenne muscular dystrophy, polymyositis has no familial tendency and can occur at any age (though it is more common in adults). Its incidence has been estimated at 5 cases per one million population per year. It is more common in the black race. Females are more frequently affected in the ratio of two to one. Initial symptoms may be abrupt, febrile and precipitated by stress. The disease follows a variable acute, subacute or chronic course which may show slow or rapid deterioration with exacerbation and remission.

Generalized proximal muscle weakness is noted (Fig. 9). When the disease is acute, muscular pain and stiffness are common (mostly in the upper extremities) and muscle calcinosis can occur. Atrophy is minimal and pseudohypertrophy occurs only occasionally. The deep tendon reflexes may be absent, normal or hyperactive. Dysphagia (due to

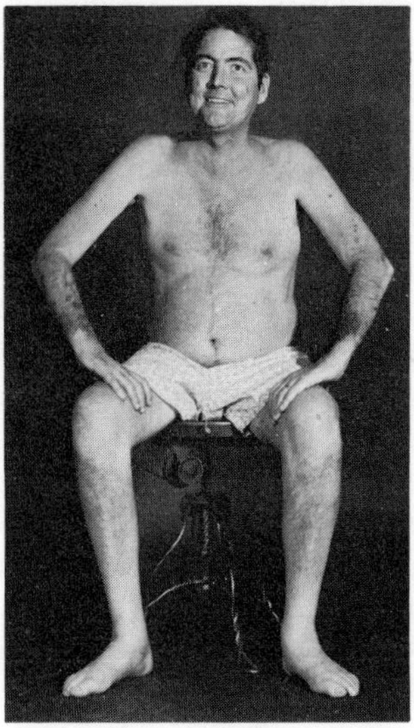

Fig. 9. Distribution of atrophy, skin rash, and edema in polymyositis.

weakness of the posterior pharyngeal muscles) is frequent. Dysphonia is sometimes heard. Intestinal hypomobility can occur as well as bowel vasculitis which can lead to perforation. The neck extensors are usually weakened.

Diagnosis is aided by an elevation of serum muscle enzymes, particularly creatinine phosphokinase, and an occasional increase in the sedimentation rate and white blood count. 50% of patients with polymyositis have a positive latex test and 50% have a rise of antinuclear antibodies. These last two parameters are normal in the patient with muscular dystrophy.

Serum electrophoresis may show elevations of Alpha 1, Alpha 2, and gamma globulin in polymyositis as in the other collagen disorders. The EMG is rarely diagnostic as an isolated test (see section on EMG). Muscle biopsy may be helpful in diagnosis (see section on Muscle Biopsy).

Adreno-cortico-steroid therapy produces dramatic results in selected cases of polymyositis. The dosage scale varies, but is usually massive (60 to 100 mg per square metre of body area) and is best given on an alternate day dosage schedule. The fluorinated steroids (dexamethasone and triamcinolone) should be avoided as they induce steroid myopathy.

Serial measurements of serum muscle enzyme are useful in assessing the effect of cortico-steroid therapy. A decline in CPK level may be seen three to four weeks prior to an increase in clinical strength. Conversely, relapses of polymyositis can be predicted some six weeks in advance of clinical weakness, as they are heralded by an increase of serum enzyme.

Long term administration of steroids is often necessary. One must plan to treat children with the disease for at least three years. Steroid myopathy superimposed upon polymyositis can occur. This is suspect if a patient shows initial improvement on steroids and then looses strength insidiously in spite of a persistent decline in serum CPK. Other features may include myalgia, cushinoid facies, and severe pelvic muscle weakness with lesser involvement of shoulder girdle and distal musculature. Steroid must be reduced in such cases. Patients are weaned from steroids slowly and carefully titrated to determine the minimal necessary maintenance dosage. Such a maintenance dosage is usually required because the treatment is suppressive, not curative, and under stress (e.g. infection) relapse of the disease may occur. Prognosis is poor for patients who are over 50 years of age, black, dysphagic, severely weakened, suffer an acute pulmonary infiltrate or have a generalized collagen disease or harbour a neoplasm.

Chart 4A. Potassium

Foods with liberal amounts of potassium are required by some people, due to certain medical treatments. The following sources (listed in order of their value) have the largest amount of potassium and are the easiest to add to the diet. These foods are also low in sodium.

Foods	*mg potassium*
½ avocado	605
* prune juice	430
5–6 dried peach halves with juice	430
½ of 4½″ cantaloupe or muskmelon	375
1 small banana	370
* orange juice, canned or fresh	365
6 medium prunes	350
** orange juice	345
* grapefruit and orange juice	335
* tangerine juice	325
** grapefruit and orange juice	320
** tangerine juice	315
** grapefruit juice	310
* blackberry juice	310
2 medium Damson plums	300
½ slice watermelon, 6″ diam. and 1½″ thick	300
* grapefruit juice, canned or fresh	295
2 medium nectarines	295
* apricot nectar	275
* tomato juice, low sodium	270
* pineapple juice	270
** pineapple juice	250
1 small tomato	245
4 canned apricot halves and 2 tbsp. juice	240
5–6 medium kumquats	235
1 oz. package of raisins	230
* grape juice	210
⅓ cup cooked rhubarb	205
⅔ cup black raspberries	200
1 small orange	200
1 medium peach	200
* apple juice	185

* 6 oz. canned juice
** concentrated juice diluted as directed, 6 oz.

Values in or calculated (rounded to the nearest 5) from COMPOSITION OF FOODS—RAW, PROCESSED, PREPARED, United States Department of Agriculture Handbook, No. 8, Revised December, 1963.

Chart 4B. 2 to 3 Gram Sodium Diet

This diet is a Full Diet with the omission of the salt shaker at table and highly salted foods. A small amount of salt may be used in cooking.

The following foods are eliminated:

Potato chips	Meat stock soups
Mustard	Gravies
Pickles	Pork
Salted nuts	Pork products
Olives	Luncheon meats
Catsup	Salted crackers

ACTH as well as immunosuppressive agents (e.g. Azothioprine, Methotrexate, Cyclophosphamide) have been used in the therapy of polymyositis. When present, a malignant neoplasm should be appropriately treated. Because prolonged administration of steroid is necessary, the usual precautions for patients on long term steroids must be taken. These include antacids, high potassium intake which may be provided through fruits containing large quantities of potassium (avocado, prunes, melons, bananas, orange juice, etc.) or KCL syrup (100 mEq. per square meter skin area daily). A low salt, low carbohydrate, isocaloric diet is advised (Chart 4). Adequate antibiotic coverage when treating concomitant infection is necessary. The patient must be closely observed for any complications to steroid therapy such as GI bleeding, cushinoid body changes, etc.

Additionally, physiatric and orthopaedic adjuncts to steroid therapy should be employed as indicated. Passive stretching of contractures, range of motion and functional strength maintaining exercising must be employed if these patients are to avoid the weakening, wasting and deformity which result from prolonged immobility. These techniques will be discussed in detail in the chapter on General Principles of Orthopaedic Treatment.

BIBLIOGRAPHY

Bohan, A. and Peter, J. B. (1975), 'Polymyositis and Dermatomyositis (Part 1),' *New Engl. J. Med.*, **292,** No. 7, 344–349.

Bohan, A. and Peter, J. B. (1975), 'Polymyositis and Dermatomyositis (Part 2),' *New Engl. J. Med.*, **292,** No. 8, 403–407.

Bonsett, C. A. (1975), 'Prophylactic Bracing in Pseudohypertrophic Muscular Dystrophy (Preliminary Report),' *J. Indiana med. Ass.*, **68,** No. 3, 181–187.

Boshes, L. D. (1967), 'Diseases of Muscles. Clinical Manifestations and Differential Diagnosis,' *New Physician*, **16,** No. 10, 263–274.

Brain, L. and Walton, J. N. (1969), *Brain's Diseases of the Nervous System*, 7th edition. London: Oxford University Press.

Caughey, J. E. and Myrianthopoulos, N. C. (1963), *Dystrophia Myotonica and Related Disorders.* Springfield, Illinois: Charles C. Thomas.

Chyatte, S. B., Rudman, D., Patterson, J. H., Gerron, Glynda G., O'Beirne, I, Barlow, Joan, Jordan, A. and Shavin, J. S. (1973), 'Human Growth Hormone and Estrogens in Boys with Duchenne Muscular Dystrophy,' *Arch. phys. med. Rehab.*, **54,** 248–253.

Dowben, R. M. (1959), 'Prolonged Survival of Dystrophic Mice Treated with 17-Ethyl-19-Nortestosterone,' *Nature*, **184,** 1966–1967.

Dubowitz, V. (1969), 'The Floppy Infant,' in *Clinics in Developmental Medicine No. 31*, England: Wm. Heinemann Medical Books Ltd. (Spastics International Medical Publications).

Dujovne, C. A. and Azarnoff, D. L. (1973), 'Clinical Complications of Corticosteroid Therapy. A Selected Review,' *Med. Clin. N. Amer.*, **57,** No. 5, 1331–1342.

Dyken, P. R. and Harper, P. S. (1973), 'Congenital Dystrophia Myotonica,' *Neurol., Minneapolis*, **23,** No. 5, 465–473.

Ford, F. F. (1966), *Diseases of the Nervous System in Infancy, Childhood and Adolescence*, 5th edition. Springfield, Illinois: Charles C. Thomas.

Girdany, B. and Danowski, T. S. (1956), 'Muscular Dystrophy,' *Amer. J. Dis. Child.*, **91,** 339–345.

Greene, R. D. (Ed.) (1969), *Myasthenia Gravis.* Philadelphia: J. B. Lippincott.

Gucker, III, T. (1971), 'Sorting out the Muscle Diseases,' *Consultant*, **II,** No. 4, 19–21.

Haas, D. C. (1973), 'Treatment of Polymyositis with Immunosuppressive Drugs,' *Neurol.*, **23,** 55–62.

Haleem, M. A. (1972), 'Myopathies in the Elderly,' *Gerontologia Clinica*, **14,** 361–377.

Harter, J. G., Reddy, W. J. and Thorn, G. W. (1963), 'Studies on an Intermittent Corticosteroid Dosage Regimen,' *New Engl. J. Med.*, **269,** 591–596.

Larsen, W. G. (1967), 'Polymyositis Dermatomyositis,' *Arch. Derm.*, **96,** 724–727.

Ludman, H. (1962), 'Dysphagia in Dystrophia Myotonica,' *J. Laryng*, **76,** 234–236.

McComas, A. J., Sica, R. E. P. and Upton, A. R. M. (1974), 'Multiple Muscle Analysis of Motor Units in Muscular Dystrophy,' *Arch. Neurol.*, **30,** 249–251.

Malpe, R. R. (Ed.), Lee, M. H. M. and Alba, A. (1973), 'Rehabilitation Technics in Polymyositis,' *N. Y. St. J. Med.*, **73,** 1208–1210.

Ogg, Elizabeth (1971), *Milestones in Muscle Disease Research.* Muscular Dystrophy Association of America, Incorporated. (Booklet published in August.)

Panayiotopoulos, C. P. and Scarpalezos, S. (1974), 'Hypertrophy of Extensor Digitorum Brevis in Limb-Girdle Muscular Dystrophy,' *Lancet*, **ii,** 230.

Patel, A. N. and Kumara, S. R. (1969), 'Muscle Percussion and Neostigmine Test in the Clinical Evaluation of Neuromuscular Disorders,' *New Eng. J. Med.*, **281,** No. 10, 523–526.

Pearn, J. H. and Wilson, J. (1973), 'Acute Werdnig-Hoffman Disease. Acute Infantile Spinal Muscular Atrophy,' *Arch. Dis. Childh.*, **48,** No. 6, 425–430.

Pearson, C. M. (1963), 'Muscular Dystrophy (Review and Recent Observations),' *Amer. J. Med.*, **35,** No. 5, 632–645.

Polgar, J. G., Bradley, W. G., Upton, A. R. M., Anderson, J., Howat, J. M. L., Petito, F., Roberts, D. F. and Scopa, J. (1972), 'The Early Detection of Dystrophia Myotonica,' *Brain*, **95,** Part IV, 761–776.

Review of Current Concepts of Myopathies. (1965), *Clinical Orthopaedics and Related Research*, No. 39. Philadelphia: J. B. Lippincott.

Scarpalezos, S. and Panayiotopoulos, C. P. (1973), 'Duchenne Muscular Dystrophy: Reservations to the Neurogenic Hypothesis,' *Lancet*, **ii,** 458.

Shy, G. M. (1962), 'The Late Onset Myopathy,' in *World Neurology*, Vol. 3, pp. 149–160.

Siegel, I. M. (1972), 'Early Signs of Landouzy-Dejerine Disease: Wrist and Finger Weakness,' *J. Amer. med. Ass.*, Letters, **221,** No. 3, 302.

Van Wijngaarden, G. K. and Bethlem, J. (1973), 'Benign Infantile Spinal Muscular Atrophy—A Prospective Study,' *Brain*, **96,** Part I, 163–170.

Walton, J. N. (Ed.) (1974), *Disorders of Voluntary Muscles*, 3rd edition. London: J. & A. Churchill, Ltd.

Welander, L. (1947), 'Neostigmine as a Diagnostic Test in Progressive Muscular Atrophy and Dystrophy,' *Acta Psychiat. (Kbh)*, suppl. 46, 329–336.

Wilner, E. C. and Brody, J. A. (1968), 'An Evaluation of the Remote Effects of Lung Cancer on the Central Nervous System,' *Neurol., Minneapolis*, **18,** No. 11, 287.

Zundel, W. S. and Tyler, F. H. (1965), 'The Muscular Dystrophies (Birth Defects Reprint Series),' *New Eng. J. Med.*, **273,** Nos. 10 and 11, 537–543, 596–601.

CHAPTER 2

Muscular Dystrophy in Young Females

Occurrence

Although recent evidence suggests that some young girls suffering from muscular dystrophy may possibly be manifesting carriers of the Duchenne gene, there is no doubt that Duchenne dystrophy, or a disease much like it can occur in young females.

Differential Diagnosis

It is rare, however, and must be carefully differentiated from benign spinal muscular atrophy of Kugelberg and Welander, a condition which often affects girls and may mimic muscular dystrophy very closely. Polymyositis must also be excluded, as well as infantile spinal muscular atrophy and severe congenital myopathy.

Findings

When this form of dystrophy occurs in a young girl, it is clinically similar to the Duchenne type, but more benign. Weakness is chiefly proximal and does not appear to differ clearly from that of Duchenne dystrophy, but progression is relatively slow. Pseudohypertrophy, particularly of the calves, is frequent (Fig. 10). Serum CPK level is only moderately elevated.

Theoretical Bases

There are a number of theoretical bases to explain the expression of an X-linked disease in girls.

1. The patient could have a Turner's syndrome (X–O gonadal dysgenesis).
2. Mating of a carrier female with an affected male (a highly unlikely possibility).
3. Mating of a carrier or normal female who has produced an ovum with a mutant X, with a normal male who has produced a sperm carrying a mutant X.
4. Lyonisation with mosaic abiotrophy. The chance inactivation of the X chromosomes in the somatic cells of the female produces a mixed population of dystrophic and non-dystrophic muscle cells. If the dystrophic cells are numerous enough, clinical symptoms appear.
5. Autosomal recessive inheritance. Such cases should be clearly distinguished from examples of limb-girdle dystrophy in consanguineous families appearing to have pseudohypertrophy as a prominent manifestation. With consanguinity of parents, autosomal recessive inheritance is likely. The late age at onset and slow rate of progression with prolonged survival differentiate these cases from typical Duchenne dystrophy.

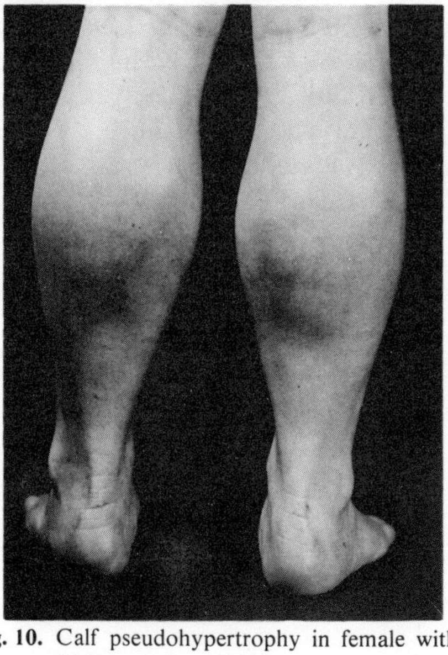

Fig. 10. Calf pseudohypertrophy in female with Duchenne dystrophy.

There is firm evidence that X-linked inheritance is characteristic of Duchenne dystrophy. This has been confirmed by the analysis of typical pedigrees and the suggestion of linkage between the gene for this form of muscular dystrophy and that of red/green (Deutane) colour blindness. It is therefore important to analyse all cases of similar disease in girls. Nonetheless, as noted above, there are theoretical reasons why an X-linked disease might appear in girls, and certainly, the practical problems of treating a clinical dystrophy in young females occasionally occurs.

BIBLIOGRAPHY

Adams, R. D., Denny-Brown, D. and Pearson, C. M. (1962), *Diseases of Muscle (A Study in Pathology)*, Hoeber Medical Book. New York: Harper & Row.

Bourne, G. H. and Golarz, M. N. (Eds.) (1963), *Muscular Dystrophy in Man and Animals*, Switzerland and New York: Publ. S. Karger, Basil.

Ionasescu, V. and Zellweger, H. (1974), 'Duchenne Muscular Dystrophy in Young Girls,' *Acta neurol. scand.*, **50,** 619–630.

Moser, H. and Emery, A. E. H. (1974), 'The Manifesting Carrier in Duchenne Muscular Dystrophy,' *Clin. Gen.*, **5,** 271–284.

Penn, Audrey S., Lisak, R. P. and Rowland, L. P. (1970), 'Muscular Dystrophy in Young Girls,' *Neurol.*, **20,** 147–159.

Symposium on Genetics of Congenital Deformity, *Clinical Orthopaedics and Related Research*, Vol. 33 (1964). Philadelphia: J. B. Lippincott.

CHAPTER 3

Serum Enzymes

Creatine-creatinine

Skeletal muscles utilize creatine and secrete creatinine in their metabolism. The reverse is true in dystrophic muscles where a decreased urinary output of creatinine and an increase in the urine creatine level are found in the symptomatic stages of the disease. There is also a lower creatine tolerance because total muscle mass is decreased. Unfortunately, these findings are not of great diagnostic significance because any disease process which significantly reduces muscle mass will increase the urinary excretion rate of creatine. This is because the reduced muscle bulk available for converting blood creatine to creatinine causes a relative increase of creatine in the blood, which exceeds its renal threshold and is excreted in the urine. This can occur with a high protein diet, starvation, carbohydrate deprivation, diabetes, wasting diseases, certain fevers, exopthalmic goitre, myasthenia gravis, various neuropathies, as well as the muscular dystrophies. There is at least one exception to this generalization and that is when blood creatine concentration is decreased in dystrophia myotonica. It is postulated that in this disease, the liver is unable to synthesize creatine at a normal rate, with subsequent decrease in its serum level.

Muscle Enzymes Available for Diagnosis in Muscle Disease

Aldolase, SGOT, SGPT

Serum aldolase is particularly abundant in skeletal muscle, but it also appears in other tissues, notably myocardium, liver and erythrocytes. Serum glutamic oxaloacetic transaminase (SGOT) and glutamic pyruvic transaminase (SGPT) are also found in skeletal muscle (SGOT more than SGPT). However, they are abundant in myocardium (where the activities of both enzymes are about 50% greater than in skeletal muscle) and in liver (where SGOT activity is similar to that in myocardium, but SGPT activity is at least ten times greater than in skeletal muscle).

These considerations indicate that serum aldolase and the transaminases are not very specific for the diagnosis of skeletal muscle disease, whether it be primary or secondary.

LDH

Lactic dehydrogenase (LDH) has been used for the diagnosis of primary muscle damage. However, its abundance (like SGOT and SGPT) in myocardium and liver, as well as in skeletal muscle, and its presence in erythrocytes, interdict its use as a specific test in the diagnosis of muscle disease. However, LDH can be fractionated electrophoretically into five bands. Studies indicate that probands as well as carriers of muscular dystrophy show an increase in bands one and two with a decrease in bands three, four and five of an LDH fractionation. The serum of patients with acute polymyositis shows an increase in bands two, three, four and five, and in chronic polymyositis bands two and five are increased.

CPK

Creatinine phosphokinase (CPK), the most specific of all muscle enzymes, provides a sensitive biochemical index for the diagnosis of diseases of skeletal muscle. It is the function of this enzyme to catalyse reversibly the transfer of an energy-rich bond from creatine phosphate to adenosine diphosphate, forming creatine and adenosine triphosphate (CRP + ADP = C + ATP). CPK can be determined by a variety of techniques. One popular method utilizes ultraviolet spectrophotometry. The normal value, of course, depends on the method used.

CPK does not appear to increase in hepatic disease and since erythrocytes contain very little CPK, hemolysis does not contaminate the analysis.

The extent of enzyme elevation depends upon the type of myopathy present, the activity of the disease, the sex of the patient, extraneous factors (such as vigorous recent exercise) and other variables. These will be listed in detail later in this chapter.

CPK elevation in the muscular dystrophies is highest in the Duchenne type and not as striking in the less rapidly progressive forms. In Duchenne muscular dystrophy serum enzyme levels are elevated early in the course of the disease. The highest levels are often found at birth and during the first year of life, well before the process is clinically evident. Because continued loss of dystrophic muscle diminishes its total efflux of enzyme, with increasing age, diminished muscle mass, and decreased functional ability, serum enzyme levels fall. Therefore, enzyme levels diminish as the disease progresses, dropping suddenly when profound atrophy portends wheelchair confinement and returning almost to normal levels in the terminal stages of the disease.

Although diagnosis of the myopathic state is usually based on clinical findings, enzyme determinations can:

1. Usually confirm the diagnosis (often before clinical findings are evident).
2. Usually distinguish between a myopathy and a neuropathy (although enzymes may be elevated in a neuropathy, such elevation is usually not as high as that found in a myopathy).
3. Occasionally differentiate certain primary myopathies from each other and from polymyositis.
4. Frequently detect a heterogenous, clinically healthy carrier of the sex-linked disease.
5. Follow the evolution and course of the myopathies (particularly the inflammatory variety), thus aiding in the evaluation of therapy and providing an index to prognosis.

Serum CPK activity is usually normal or only slightly elevated in patients with muscular weakness of neurogenic origin. However, some chronic denervating diseases may simulate myopathy with markedly elevated CPK. In patients with primary disease of muscle, enzyme activities are raised, sometimes grossly. These elevations in the patient with minimal muscle weakness without other evident disease are a very strong indication of the presence of a myopathy.

The clinical course in the adult forms of muscular dystrophy may be variable so that the rate of muscle loss in inconstant. Thus, serum CPK levels cannot correlate well with duration of the illness because elevation of CPK and the magnitude of its variations are proportional to the remaining mass of dystrophic muscle and severity of the disease. One, therefore, finds serum enzyme elevations at variations greater in early than in late Duchenne type dystrophy, less striking in the limb-girdle and facioscapulohumeral types and least prominent in myotonic diseases.

The 'normal range' of CPK is affected by age (higher in ages 10 to 19 and 40 to 49), race (higher in blacks than in white) and physical activity (higher after exercise). Other conditions causing CPK* elevation are as follows:

1. Myocardial infarction.
2. Intramuscular injection.
3. Alcoholism.
4. Muscular injury.
5. Malignant hyperthermia.
6. Subarachnoid hemorrhage.
7. Brain tumour.
8. Convulsions.
9. Meningitis.
10. Encephalitis.
11. Acute psychosis.
12. Hypokalemia.
13. A variety of acute abdominal conditions (e.g. hemorrhagic pancreatitis, gangrene of the gallbladder).

CPK lability is reflected in the higher level noted in out-patients vs. inpatients and in its elevation (usually slight) in some neuropathies (e.g. Charcot-Marie tooth disease).

Serum enzyme levels are elevated in polymyositis and, as one might expect, the degree of elevation depends upon the rate of progression, degree of weakness and severity of the inflammation. In fulminating in-

* There are at least three isoenzymes of CPK, one concentrated largely in the central nervous system, one in skeletal muscle and another in cardiac muscle.

Chart 5 CPK Elevations, Signs, Symptoms, and other Findings in Diseases with Muscle Weakness

Disease	*CPK*	*Family History*	*Pseudohypertrophy*	*Remission or non-progression*	*Fasciculation and Fibrillation*
Duchenne muscular dystrophy:					
Early in course	++++	++++	++++	0	±
Late in course	++	++++	++	0	0
Late onset variant	++++	++++	++++	0	±
Limb-girdle muscular dystrophy:					
Early onset	++	+	0	0	0
Late onset	+	+	0	0	0
Fascioscapulohumeral dystrophy	+	++	+	0	0
Myotonic dystrophy	±	+++	0	0	Myotonia
Acute myositis	+++	0	0	++++	+
Polymyositis	++	+	+	++	+
Benign muscular hypotonia	Normal	+	0	+++	0
Thyrotoxic myopathies	±	0	0	++	0
Spinal muscular atrophy	Normal	+	0	0	++++
Peripheral polyneuropathies	±	0	0	++	++
Amyotrophic lateral sclerosis	Normal	0	0	0	Fasciculations

(Adapted from Coodley, E. L. (Ed.) (1970), *Diagnostic Enzymology*, Philadelphia, Pennsylvania: Lea & Febinger, Chap. 9, p. 263.)

flammatory muscle disease CPK levels are often very high (more than five times normal), whereas in persons with indolent disease, elevations of several times normal usually are found.

Serial CPK determinations may be used to monitor the effectiveness of steroid therapy in polymyositis. During the administration of steroids, decline in the serum enzyme level anticipates clinical improvement; conversely, when the steroid dosage is being reduced, a rise in enzyme level presages a decrease in muscle strength. Thus, the progress of a patient can be followed by serial measurement which is helpful in adjusting the steroid dosage necessary to treat any stage of the disease.

Chart 5 tabulates relative elevations of serum CPK enzyme activity correlated with several other significant diagnostic parameters in a variety of diseases presenting with muscular weakness.

BIBLIOGRAPHY

Bourne, G. H. (1972), *The Structure and Function of Muscle*, 2nd edition, Vol. 1. New York and London: Academic Press.

Coodley, E. L. (Ed.) (1970), *Diagnostic Enzymology.* Philadelphia, Pennsylvania: Lea & Febiger.

Goto, I. (1974), 'Creatine Phosphokinase Isozymes in Neuromuscular Disorders,' *Arch. Neurol.*, **31,** 116–119.

Munsat, T. L., Baloh, R., Pearson, C. M. and Fowler, W., Jr. (1973), 'Serum Enzyme Alterations in Neuromuscular Disorders,' *J. Amer. med. Ass.*, **226,** No. 13, 1536–1543.

Murphy, E. G. (1964), *The Chemistry and Therapy of Disorders of Voluntary Muscles.* Springfield, Illinois: Charles C. Thomas.

Nevins, M. A., Saran, M., Bright, M. and Lyon, L. J. (1973). 'Pitfalls in Interpreting Serum Creatine Phosphokinase Activity,' *J. Amer. med. Ass.*, **224,** No. 10, 1382–1387.

Telford, Ira Wood (1971), *Experimental Muscular Dystrophies in Animals (A Comparative Study).* Springfield, Illinois: Charles C. Thomas.

Zellweger, J. and Antonik, A. *Newborn Screening for Duchenne Muscular Dystrophy.* Muscular Dystrophy Associations of America, Inc., National Institutes of Health, USPHS Clinical Research Center, Grant MO1 FR 59, and State Services for Crippled Children Special Project Budget MR 12, HEW.

CHAPTER 4

Detection of the Carrier State

Genetic counselling is an important part of the total treatment of a patient with muscular dystrophy. Although approximately one third of all cases of Duchenne dystrophy are sporadic neomutations, mothers of afflicted children should know if they are carriers of the disease, so that future pregnancies can be planned. In addition, sisters of such patients have to be tested for the carrier state and counselled concerning the risk of having a child with muscular dystrophy. As a general rule, dominant traits are less severe than recessive ones. This is because dominant lethal traits disappear and dominant non-lethal genes tend to be structural abnormalities or changes in nonenzyme proteins, whereas recessively inherited traits tend to be inborn metabolic errors or enzyme defects.

For a woman to be a carrier of the gene for one of the X-linked dystrophies there is a 50% chance that any male child will be affected, and a 50% chance that any female child will be born a carrier of the

Table 1 Consultand with an Affected *Brother*, N1 Normal Brothers and N2 Normal Sons. It is Assumed that two-thirds of Known Carriers have C.P.K. Levels Greater than the Normal 95 Percentile (N).

C.P.K.		*Normal sons* (N2)				*Normal brothers* (N1)								
Consultand	Consultand's Mother	0	1	2	3	0	1	2	3	4	5	6	7	8
		+				0.3333	0.2500	0.1667	0.1000	0.0556	0.0294	0.0152	0.0077	0.0039
			+			0.2000	0.1429	0.0909	0.0526	0.0286	0.0149	0.0076	0.0039	0.0019
				+		0.1111	0.0769	0.0476	0.0270	0.0145	0.0075	0.0038	0.0019	0.0010
					+	0.0588	0.0400	0.0244	0.0137	0.0073	0.0038	0.0019	0.0010	0.0005
N		+				0.1493	0.1047	0.0656	0.0375	0.0202	0.0105	0.0054	0.0027	0.0014
			+			0.0806	0.0552	0.0339	0.0191	0.0102	0.0053	0.0027	0.0014	0.0007
				+		0.0420	0.0284	0.0172	0.0097	0.0051	0.0027	0.0013	0.0007	0.0003
					+	0.0215	0.0144	0.0087	0.0048	0.0026	0.0013	0.0007	0.0003	0.0002
N	N	+				0.0835	0.0498	0.0275	0.0145	0.0075	0.0038	0.0019	0.0018	0.0005
			+			0.0436	0.0255	0.0140	0.0073	0.0038	0.0019	0.0018	0.0005	0.0002
				+		0.0223	0.0129	0.0070	0.0037	0.0019	0.0018	0.0005	0.0002	0.0001
					+	0.0113	0.0065	0.0035	0.0018	0.0009	0.0005	0.0002	0.0001	0.1001

Table 1 (*contd.*) Consultand with an Affected *Son*, N1 Normal Brothers and N2 Normal Sons. It is Assumed that two-thirds of Known Carriers have C.P.K. Levels Greater than the Normal 95 Percentile (N).

C.P.K.		*Normal sons* (N2)				*Normal brothers* (N1)								
Consultand	Consultand's Mother	0	1	2	3	0	1	2	3	4	5	6	7	8
		+				0.6667	0.6000	0.5556	0.5294	0.5152	0.5077	0.5039	0.5019	0.5010
			+			0.5000	0.4286	0.3846	0.3600	0.3469	0.3402	0.3368	0.3351	0.3342
				+		0.3333	0.2727	0.2381	0.2195	0.2099	0.2050	0.2029	0.2012	0.2006
					+	0.2000	0.1579	0.1351	0.1233	0.1172	0.1142	0.1127	0.1119	0.1115
N		+				0.4124	0.3448	0.3049	0.2830	0.2716	0.2657	0.2627	0.2612	0.2605
			+			0.2597	0.2083	0.1799	0.1648	0.1571	0.1532	0.1512	0.1502	0.1497
				+		0.1493	0.1163	0.0988	0.0898	0.0853	0.0830	0.0818	0.0812	0.0809
					+	0.0806	0.0617	0.0520	0.0470	0.0445	0.0433	0.0426	0.0423	0.0422
N	N	+				0.3216	0.2920	0.2762	0.2681	0.2639	0.2618	0.2608	0.2603	0.2600
			+			0.1916	0.1710	0.1602	0.1548	0.1520	0.1506	0.1499	0.1496	0.1494
				+		0.1059	0.0935	0.0871	0.0839	0.0823	0.0815	0.0811	0.0808	0.0807
					+	0.0559	0.0490	0.0455	0.0438	0.0429	0.0425	0.0422	0.0421	0.0421

See explanation overleaf

Table 1. This table demonstrates the chances of a consultand being a carrier of Duchenne muscular dystrophy. The term 'consultand' refers to the female seeking genetic advice with either an affected brother or an affected son (both situations are covered in separate sections of the table). The figures are for suspect females who have normal CPK's. If the CPK is elevated, the individual is by definition a carrier and the table does not apply.

In addition to the number of normal brothers and normal sons, the table also considers whether the consultand's mother has a normal CPK level or whether the CPK has not been determined either on herself or her mother (indicated by blank spaces in the appropriate columns).

If the consultand's CPK is half the upper level of normal, then the probability is decreased by one-half the indicated value. It can be proportionally reduced further depending upon the specific CPK value. Probability statistics are presented as decimals.

As an example, if a mother has a single affected son, a normal CPK, three normal sons and two normal brothers, and her mother's CPK is not available, the chances of her being a carrier of Duchenne muscular dystrophy would be .052 (slightly over 5%) and the odds of her having an affected son are one-fourth of this.

This data is reproduced through the kind permission of Professor Alan E. H. Emery, Department of Human Genetics, Western General Hospital, Edinburgh, Scotland (Emery, A. E. H. *et al.*, 1967, *Genetic Counselling in Muscular Dystrophy*, In Proc. IInd International Congress of Neuro-genetics and Neuro-ophthalmology, pp. 106–110, Excerpta Medica International Congress Series No. 175, Amsterdam).

condition*. However, bayesian statistics indicate that as a carrier mother has normal male children, her chances of having a son with the disease are less (Table 1). The risk of a daughter whose CPK is normal, whose mother's CPK is normal, and whose brother has Duchenne muscular dystrophy is only one to 52 that she will give birth to a dystrophic son. If, however, her mother has an elevated CPK, even though her own CPK is normal, that risk rises to one to sixteen. The risk of a sporadic occurrence of Duchenne muscular dystrophy is one in 4000. If the maternal grandfather is over 35 years of age at the time of the mother's birth, there is an increased chance of that mother being a carrier. Finally, if a single affected male represents a sporadic mutation, there is a one in three chance that the mother is normal and will not have another male child with muscular dystrophy.

Women 'at risk' may be categorized as follows:

1. **Definite carriers.** Those who are mothers of an affected son who also have an affected brother, maternal uncle, sister's son, or other dystrophic male relatives in the female line of inheritance, or who are mothers of affected sons by different nonconsanguineous fathers.

2. **Probable carriers.** Mothers of two or more sons with muscular dystrophy who have no other affected relatives.

3. **Possible carriers.** Mothers of isolated cases, and sisters and other female relatives of affected males. Such possible carriers may have a known risk (e.g. a daughter of a definite carrier where the risk is 50%), or an unknown risk (the sister of a sporadic case).

As the genetics become progressively more obscure, so does the prognosis for an individual couple improve because, as a general rule, every complication of the simple Mendelian scheme lowers the probability of transmitting an abnormal gene.

The most sensitive serum enzyme for detection of the carrier state is creatine phosphokinase. This fact has been confirmed in large series of relatives of patients with Duchenne dystrophy. However, the test provides less useful information in relatives of patients afflicted with any of the three less acute, usually autosomal hereditary forms of dystrophy (limb-girdle, facioscapulohumeral, dystrophia myotonica).

* Duchenne dystrophics do not survive to reproduce. In benign X-linked (Becker) dystrophy, affected males may survive into adulthood and have children. All sons born to such a father will be normal and all his daughters will be carriers.

Identification of carriers depends upon the fact that they carry a microcosm of the disease which may be detected by appropriate investigation. In the case of muscular dystrophy carriers, close physical examination will often reveal slight weakness of the limb-girdle musculature and even calf enlargement. Indeed, some young females apparently suffering from muscular dystrophy may be manifesting carriers of the disease.

Because of the degradation occurring in the cells representing this limited myopathy, detection of the carrier state by discovery of an elevated serum CPK is usually more accurate during childhood. By the time many carriers reach adulthood (or even late adolescence), all myopathic cells have fully degraded, and serum CPK has returned to normal. The very best time to test for elevated CPK is before age 10, which is also the time it begins to decrease in the average Duchenne dystrophic.

On the other hand, neonatal CPK levels are sometimes elevated, and this increase in serum enzyme, reflecting both birth trauma and extremely active neonatal muscle metabolism, may persist into early infancy. It is wise to delay CPK determination for detection of the carrier state until at least one year of age.

A minimal elevation of CPK may present as a benign variant in otherwise normal individuals (including unaffected brothers or patients with Duchenne dystrophy), and CPK may be slightly elevated in 'normal' individuals after physical activity. The 'normal range' is affected by age, race, and sex. CPK is normally higher in the evening and in the winter (this reflects a circadian rhythm pattern). Elevated CPK has been noted in a wide variety of disease states. This matter is elaborated upon in the section on laboratory diagnosis by serum enzyme determination.

In spite of these limitations, careful biochemical screening should allow detection of over 75% of all carriers of Duchenne dystrophy. Other sometimes useful methods of detecting the carrier state are as follows:

1. Abnormality of beta globulin fraction of serum proteins.
2. Decrease in total body potassium.
3. Increase of muscle fraction of LDH isoenzymes.
4. Positive muscle biopsy.
5. Changes in electrophysiology of muscle, including:
    a. Measurement of absolute refractory period of muscle fibres.

b. Measurement of the duration and number of phases of motor unit action potentials.
c. Analysis of the interference pattern by use of an automatic spike counter and computer.
Note: All the above require quantitative EMG.

6. Elevated polyribosome protein synthesis.
7. EKG changes resembling cardiomyopathy of Duchenne dystrophy.

By using CPK determinations* and these techniques when necessary, successful detection of 90% of carriers should be possible.

The congenital risk factor for the 'normal' population at large is 3% for any given pregnancy. Female carriers of muscular dystrophy should be counselled regarding the risk inherent in their pregnancies. If they choose to have their own children, it may be possible to identify fetal sex by the sixteenth to twentieth week of pregnancy by amniocentesis, and therapeutic abortion performed if the fetal cells indicate a male chromosomal pattern. However, if only such male children are aborted and the females allowed to come to term, more carriers will inevitably be born. Under these circumstances there is an increased chance of the family forgetting or denying a carrier of muscular dystrophy in its pedigree, and ultimately the population of children with Duchenne muscular dystrophy will increase rather than decrease.

By far the best course to be followed is for all known carriers of Duchenne muscular dystrophy to avoid pregnancy and adopt children if they desire a family.

BIBLIOGRAPHY

Emery, A. E. H. (1969), 'Genetic Counselling in X-linked Muscular Dystrophy,' in *Journal of the Neurological Sciences*, Vol. 8, pp. 579–587. Amsterdam: Elsevier Publishing Company.

Emery, A. E. H. (1964), 'Electrophoretic Pattern of Lactic Dehydrogenase in Carriers and Patients with Duchenne Muscular Dystrophy,' *Nature*, **201,** 1044–1045.

Fowler, W. M., Gardner, G. W., Taylor, R. G., Scavarda, A. and Busheikin, J. B. (1969), 'Quantitative Measurements in Female Siblings and Mothers of Boys with Duchenne Dystrophy,' *Arch. phys. Med. Rehab.*, **50,** 301–310.

* CPK should be measured on three separate days and an average value determined.

Ionassescu, V., Zellweger, H., Shirk, P. and Conway, T. W. (1973), 'Identification of Carriers of Duchenne Muscular Dystrophy by Muscle Protein Synthesis,' *Neurol., Minneapolis*, **23,** No. 5, 497–502.

Mann, O., DeLeon, A. C., Jr., Perloff, J. K., Simanis, J. and Horrigan, F. D. (from the Department of Medicine, Division of Cardiology, Geogetown University School of Medicine, Washington, D.C.) (1968), 'Duchenne's Muscular Dystrophy: The Electrocardiogram in Female Relatives,' *Amer. J. med. Sci.*, **255,** 376–381.

Pearn, J. H. (1973), 'Patients: Subjective Interpretation of Risks Offered in Genetic Counselling, *J. med. Gen.*, **10,** No. 2, 129–134.

Skinner, Rosalind and Emery, A. E. H. (1974), 'Serum-Creatine-Kinase Levels in Carriers of Becker Muscular Dystrophy,' *Lancet*, **ii,** 1023–1024.

CHAPTER 5

Muscle Biopsy

Conditions for Muscle Biopsy
Technique
Site
Value of Biopsy
Differential Histopathology
Neuropathy
Myopathy
Polymyositis
Histochemistry

Biopsy is an important tool in the diagnosis of muscle disease. However, the site of biopsy must be carefully chosen. The muscle selected should be only moderately involved clinically. A muscle graded at 2 or 3 is best.* Choosing a muscle that is not at all involved, or a muscle that has been totally destroyed decreases the value of biopsy. In early disease choose a weak muscle, in later disease one relatively strong. Muscle which has recently been traumatized by needle penetration from electromyography should not be biopsied as such testing produces histological artifacts.

The biopsy should be well planned with all necessary solutions for biochemical and histochemical studies available. If local anaesthesia is used, one must avoid direct trauma to the muscle under biopsy by the needle or by infiltration of muscle tissue with the anaesthetic agent.

* The following key for grading muscle strength is employed:

5. Complete range of motion against gravity with full resistance.
4. Complete range of motion against gravity with some resistance.
3. Complete range of motion against gravity.
2. Complete range of motion with gravity eliminated.
1. Evidence of slight contractility. No joint motion.
0. No evidence of contractility.

Muscle removed for histologic examination should be kept at its original *in situ* length. This can best be accomplished by using one of several special biopsy clamps available (Fig. 11). The muscle is sectioned on either side of the clamp and placed directly in a solution of glutaraldehyde to terminate enzymatic activity. After one hour, the biopsy specimen, still clamped, is transferred to freshly buffered formalin solution. Special techniques are available for nerve detail, as well as special fixation processes for electron-microscopy.

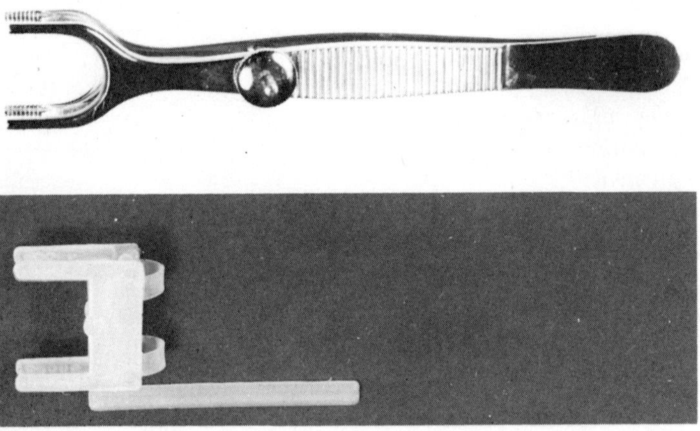

Fig. 11. Two types of muscle biopsy clamps designed to keep the specimen at its original *in situ* length. The one pictured below is made of disposable plastic.

Removal of several adjacent superficial strips of muscle is preferable to biopsy of tissue located deep within the muscle bundle. Careful, sharp dissection is mandatory to avoid hematoma. It is unnecessary to take a massive specimen.

The gastrocnemius is usually a poor muscle for biopsy. If the lower limb is favoured, the vastus lateralis is often the best muscle available for biopsy. Ordinarily, the rectus abdominus is the preferred site, as it is usually in the early stage of involvement, and biopsy here does not even minimally impair ambulation.

A well performed and expertly interpreted muscle biopsy can usually distinguish a neuropathy from a myopathy, often diagnose an inflammatory myopathy, and frequently differentiate the congenital myopathies. (The diagnosis of mitochondral myopathy requires an electron microscope. The other congenital myopathies can often be diagnosed by light microscopy.)

Muscle biopsy cannot be used for purposes of determining prognosis, assessing degree of involvement or evaluating therapy. It is also impossible by standard biopsy alone* to distinguish between the common muscular dystrophies (Duchenne, limb-girdle, FSH, dystrophia myotonica).

The classical histopathological findings differentiating neuropathy from myopathy are as follows (Figs. 12 and 13):

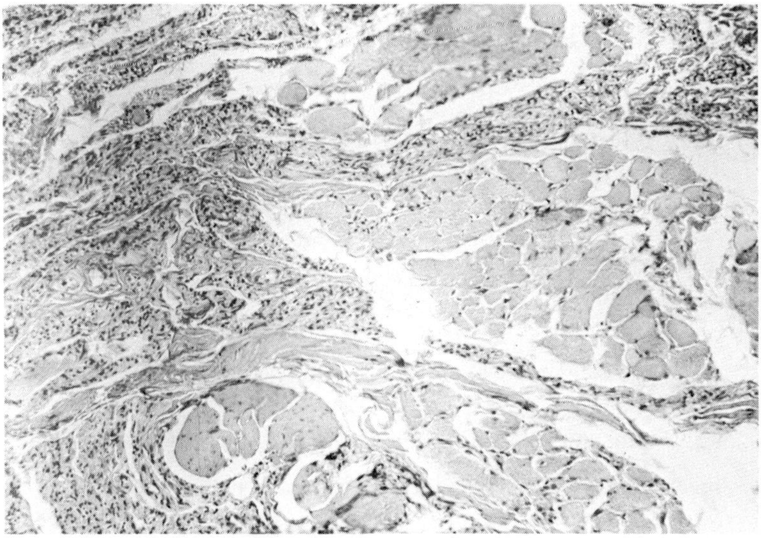

Fig. 12. Neuropathic atrophy.

Neuropathic atrophy

1. Small fibres on cross section.
2. Bundles of atrophic small fibres interspersed with bundles of normal sized, normally innervated fibres.
3. Little increase in connective tissue.

Myopathic atrophy

1. Fibre necrosis, preceded by swelling and loss of cross striations.

* Some histochemical and/or electron microscopic differences may exist.

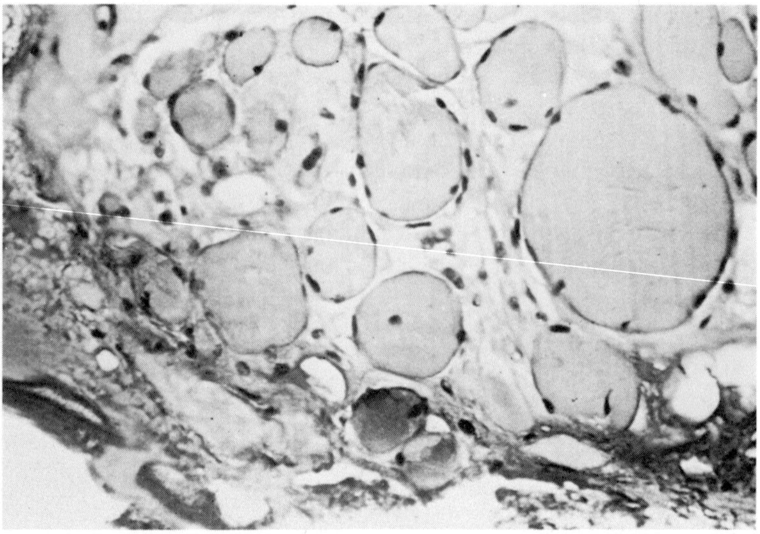

Fig. 13. Myopathic atrophy.

2. Deposition of fat and connective tissue proliferation.
3. Hyaline, granular and fatty degeneration.
4. Increased number of nuclei and nuclear migration to centre of muscle fibres.
5. Finding of enlarged nuclei enclosing large nucleoli.

Aggregates of inflammatory cells are seen in polymyositis (Fig. 14). However, cellular evidence of inflammation is also often seen in the early stages of Duchenne dystrophy. Other histopathological findings in polymyositis include:

1. Segmental necrosis.
2. Fibre degeneration and regeneration.
3. Interstitial edema and/or fibrosis.
4. Phagocytosis of necrotic fibres.
5. Perivasculitis.
6. Perifascicular muscle fibre atrophy.

Finally, a variety of histochemical techniques are available for diagnosis. These tests, though lacking the precision of quantitative biochemical methods, permit anatomical localization of enzymes and other materials. They are valuable in diagnosing such conditions as

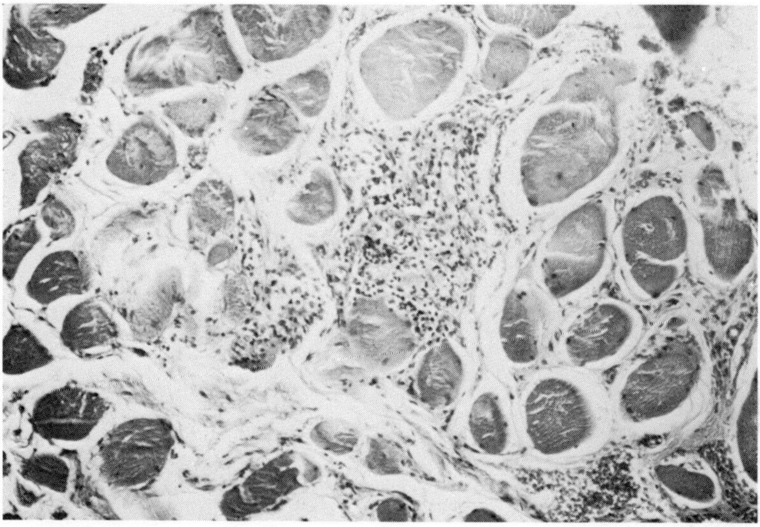

Fig. 14. Polymyositis.

glycogen-storage disease and certain exotic myopathies (i.e. central core disease), and in revealing certain features of microscopic anatomy (i.e. fibre type). However, these techniques are usually only available in the research oriented hospital.

BIBLIOGRAPHY

Banker, B. Q. (Ed.) (1972), *Research in Muscle Development and the Muscle Spindle*. Exerpta Medica Foundation.

Dubowitz, V. and Brooke, M. H. (1973), *Muscle Biopsy: A Modern Approach*. England: W. B. Saunders Company Ltd.

Greenfield, J. G., Shy, G. M., Alvord, E. C., Jr. and Berg, L. (1957), *An Atlas of Muscle Pathology in Neuromuscular Diseases*. Edinburgh and London: Livingstone.

Milhorat, A. T. (Ed.) (1967), *Exploratory Concepts in Muscular Dystrophy and Related Disorders*. Exerpta Medica Foundation.

Rayport, M. (1969), 'A Disposable Isometric Muscle Biopsy Clamp,' *J. Amer. med. Ass.*, **210,** No. 8, 1451–1452.

CHAPTER 6

Electromyography (EMG)

Technique and Use

The use of EMG has proved valuable in the diagnosis of muscle disease. It is an examination which is relatively simple and well tolerated by most patients. It is, however, not entirely reliable in unco-operative youngsters. The EMG must be conducted by a skilled electromyographer. Single motor unit potentials are elicited and interpreted. Normal muscle is usually electrically silent at rest, except for insertional activity secondary to needle stimulation, and occasional fasciculation (normal myokymia).

EMG is useful in differentiating diseases of the anterior horn cell, peripheral nerve,* and muscle. Important components to be interpreted include:

1. Amplitude.
2. Frequency.
3. Duration of the summed action potentials on sample of a population of muscle fibres (Fig. 15).

* Nerve conduction velocity studies are useful in distinguishing anterior horn cell disease from pathology in the peripheral nerve.

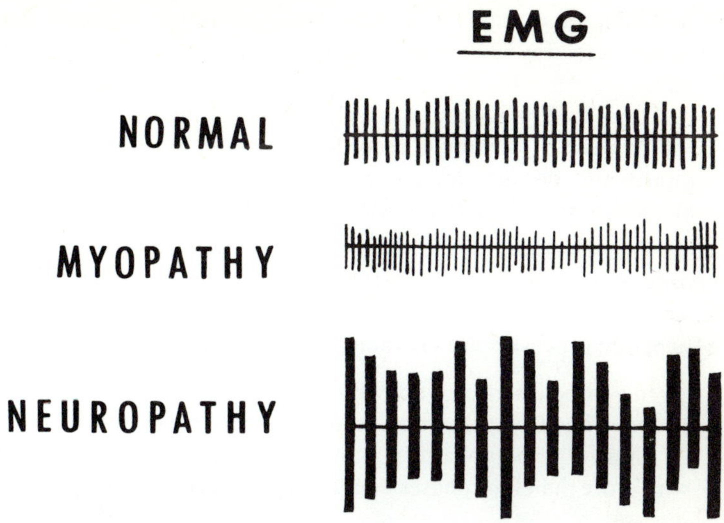

Fig. 15. Schematic diagram of features of electrical response in EMG for (1) normal, (2) myopathic (increased frequency, decreased duration, decreased amplitude), and (3) neuropathic (decreased frequency, increased duration, increased amplitude) states. (Modified from *Chicago Medicine*, 11 August, 1973, by courtesy of N. A. Vick, M.D. and the Chicago Medical Society.)

Characteristics

The major EMG features of a neuropathic process are:

1. Frequent fibrillation potentials—spontaneous discharges of single muscle fibre occurring in the absence of voluntary muscular contraction. This is a sign of denervation. However, fibrillation potentials can also occur in myopathy because of secondary terminal nerve involvement from connective tissue changes.
2. Group polyphasic potentials—muscle action potentials with more than four phases, occurring as groups.
3. Reduced interference pattern—pattern of overlapping potentials produced during a maximal muscle contraction. Reduced and overlapping in neurogenic disease.
4. Increased amplitude of muscle potential—an increase in electrical activity, recorded from the muscle fibres of a motor unit due to re-innervation of muscle fibres by the sprouting of uninvolved nerve cell processes.

5. Increased duration of muscle action potential—a longer time of electrical activity recorded from the muscle fibres of a motor unit.
6. Decreased frequency of muscle action potential—a decrease in the number of potentials recorded from the muscle fibres of a motor unit because fewer units are available for firing, having atrophied secondary to disease of the motor neuron.

Thus, neuropathies are characterized by *decreased frequency*, *increased amplitude*, and *increased duration* of electrical activity (Fig. 16).

Myopathic processes are characterized on the EMG by:

1. Increased insertional activity—increase in the electrical activity occurring during insertion or movement of the needle electrode.
2. Short-type polyphasic potentials—a muscle action potential with more than four phases does not appear grouped in myopathic disease.
3. Retained interference pattern—a pattern of overlapping potential produced during a maximal muscle contraction. No reduced overlapping occurs in myopathic disorders.
4. Reduced amplitude of muscle action potential—a reduction in the size of electrical activity is recorded from the muscle fibres of a motor unit because scattered fibres within the sampled field are not functioning.
5. Reduced duration of muscle action potential—a shorter time of electrical activity recorded from the muscle fibres of a motor unit.

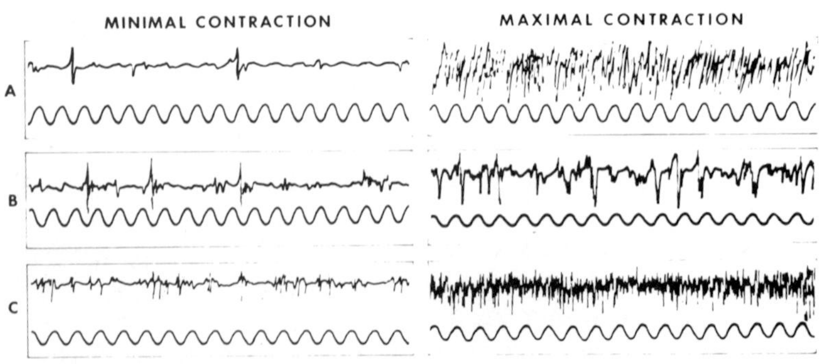

Fig. 16. EMG in (a) normal, (b) neuropathic, and (c) myopathic muscle. (Modified from *Disorders of Voluntary Muscle*, 3rd Edn. (1974) by courtesy of J. N. Walton, M.D. (Ed.) and Churchill Livingstone.)

6. Increased frequency of muscle action potential—an increase in the number of potentials recorded from the muscle fibres of a motor unit because more such units are called upon to support muscle contraction.

Thus, a typical EMG in a myopathy shows *increased frequency* but *decreased amplitude* and *decreased duration* of electrical activity, recorded from the muscle fibres of a motor unit (Fig. 16).

The characteristic EMG in dystrophia myotonica is a combination of myotonic insertion activity (many trains of spiked potentials and positive waves fired at a high frequency which then wax and wane until they die out). The 'dive bomber' sound of these myotonic potentials is specific for myotonia.

The presence of myopathic, rather than normal motor unit potentials, is the essential difference between dystrophia myotonica and myotonia congenita, an important distinction because prognosis in these conditions is vastly different.

The EMG in polymyositis combines neuropathic and myopathic features. The changes are essentially quantitative and include:

1. Prolonged insertional activity.
2. Short duration action potentials.
3. Positive sharp waves.
4. A complex polyphasic electric pattern with greatly reduced amplitude on voluntary contraction of the muscle.
5. Spontaneous fibrillation potentials, indistinguishable from denervation fibrillation, occurring at complete rest or after mild mechanical stimulation of the muscle.
6. Groups of repetitive potentials of very brief duration, resembling very closely the 'dive bomber' sound of the myotonic phenomenon, except that they are much less intense and fade more slowly.

Study of the electrical activity of skeletal muscle does not by itself always supply a diagnosis. However, it can indicate whether the lower motor neuron or the muscle is the site of a lesion and sometimes even categorize the disease process more specifically within that anatomy.

BIBLIOGRAPHY

Swaiman, K. L. and Wright, F. S. (1970), *Neuro-muscular Diseases of Infancy and Childhood*, Springfield, Illinois: Charles C. Thomas.

Symposium on Muscular Skeletal Disorders, Vol. 14, No. 2 (1967). Pediatric Clinics of North America.

Vick, N. A. (1973), 'Disease of Skeletal Muscle—Current Ideas of Diagnosis and Management,' *Chicago Med.*, **76,** No. 16, 621–625.

CHAPTER 7

X-Ray

Roentgen Features of Muscular Dystrophy
Osteoporosis
Talipes Equinocavovarus
Vertebral Caninization
Decreased Tibial Diameter
Overtubulation of Long Bone Shafts
Symmetric Diminution in Scapular Size
Small Pelvis, Flaring Iliac Bones, Prominent Ischial Spines
Increased Soft Tissue Shadow
Hip Valgus
Lordosis, Scoliosis
Roentgen Features of Dystrophia Myotonia
GI Dysfunction
Skull Changes
Pulmonary Disease

Roentgen features in muscular dystrophy, though not pathognomonic of the disease, include:

1. **Osteoporosis.** This is a late change in advanced disease due to muscular enfeeblement and disuse. Epiphyses sometimes have a radiolucent centre surrounded by a peripheral, thin, dense line (signet ring appearance), while the remainder of the bone shows profound demineralization (Fig. 17).

2. **Talipes equinocavovarus.** This, as well as other contractures, is found in the advanced stages of dystrophy, secondary to abnormal posture due to unopposed muscle contraction (Fig. 18).

3. **Vertebral caninization.** An increase in relative altitude of the

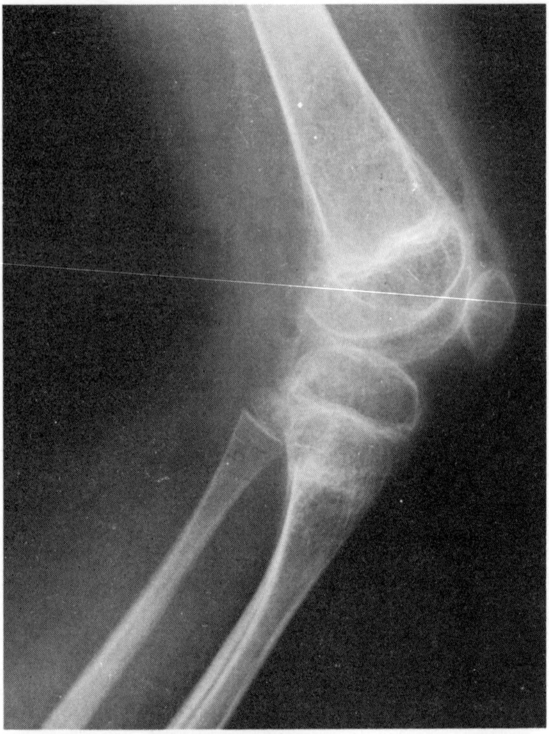

Fig. 17.

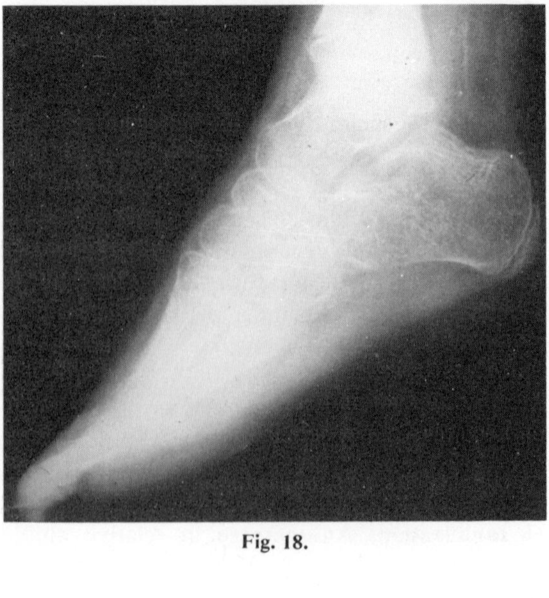

Fig. 18.

vertebral bodies (which may ultimately be as high as they are wide), as in the quadruped. This nonspecific change is seen in children chronically bedridden for any cause (Fig. 19).

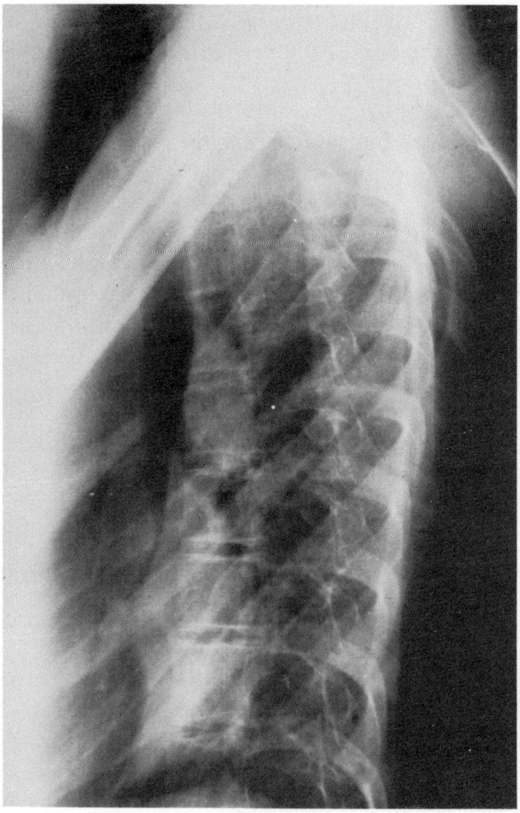

Fig. 19.

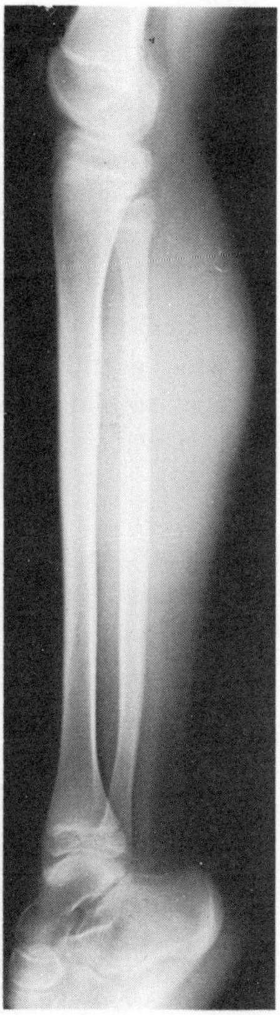

Fig. 20.

4. Decreased tibial diameter. Accompanied by increased AP fibular thickness (on lateral view), with decreased (transverse) frontal fibular diaphysial diameter. Due to a lack of normal growth stimulation secondary to muscular tension. Found in the childhood myopathies. A lateral X-ray will often show the width of the middle third of the tibial diaphysis to be no larger than that of the adjacent fibula. Linear growth (enchondral) is not as much affected as circumferential growth (membranous) in the long bones because circumferential growth depends upon normal muscle function (Fig. 20).

5. Overtubulation of long bone shafts. Occurs with early onset of muscular dystrophy. Long bones become thin with decrease in the diaphyseal cortex and narrowing of the medullary canal (concentric atrophy) (Fig. 21).

6. Symmetric diminution in the size of the scapulae. This is found in dystrophies of childhood onset.

7. Small pelvis with flaring iliac bones and prominent ischial spines. Such changes are noted when a child is confined early to a wheelchair (Fig. 22).

8. Increased soft tissue shadow (in areas of hypertrophy and pseudohypertrophy). With hypertrophy, the soft tissue density is that of muscle, but with pseudohypertrophy it becomes striated with shadows of fat density secondary to fatty infiltration. This is a late phenomenon (Fig. 23).

9. Valgus hip deformity (femoral neck angle often greater than 140°). Again, due to lack of muscle tension about the hip (Fig. 24).

10. Lordosis (early) and scoliosis (late). See sections on Pathomechanics and Scoliosis for full explanation of these phenomena.

11. Roentgen findings described in dystrophia myotonica include:

a. Esophageal dysfunction, inability to swallow a normal sized bolus, poor peristalsis and laryngeal spilling from the pharynx.
b. Colonic atony on barium enema.
c. Changes in the skull, including a small sella tursica, hyperostosis frontalis, leontiasis ossea, large frontal sinuses, and poor mandibular angle.
d. Elevation of the diaphragm secondary to phrenic nerve atrophy.
e. Finally, basal atelectasis and pneumonitis (a frequent cause of death in muscular dystrophy) can be noted in advanced cases. Cardiomyopathy (enlargement) may be recognized roentgenographically, but EKG is a better test in this regard.

All of the bone changes seen in the myopathies occur because of muscular weakness, atrophy and/or contracture. They do not express a basic mesodermal defect.

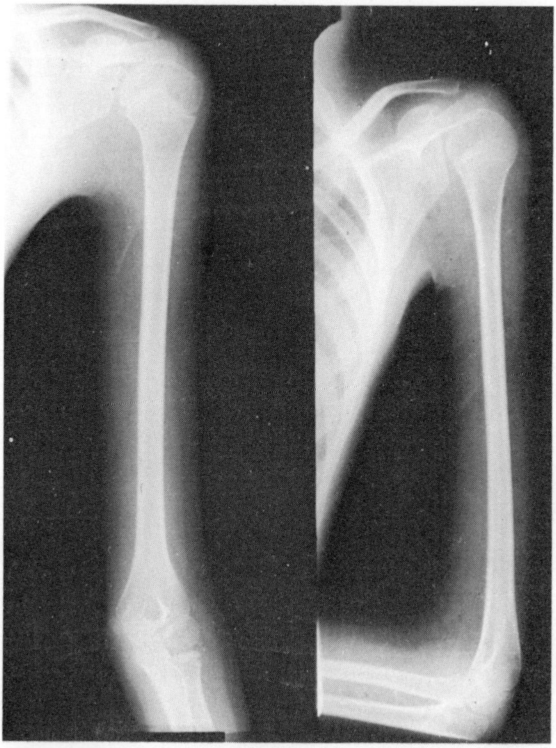

Fig. 21.

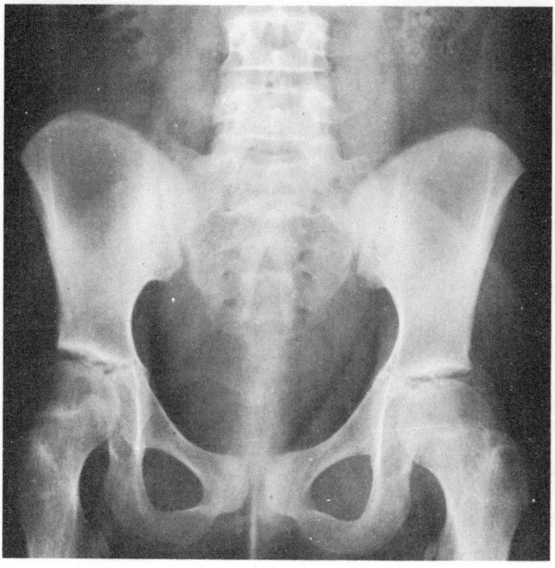

Fig. 22.

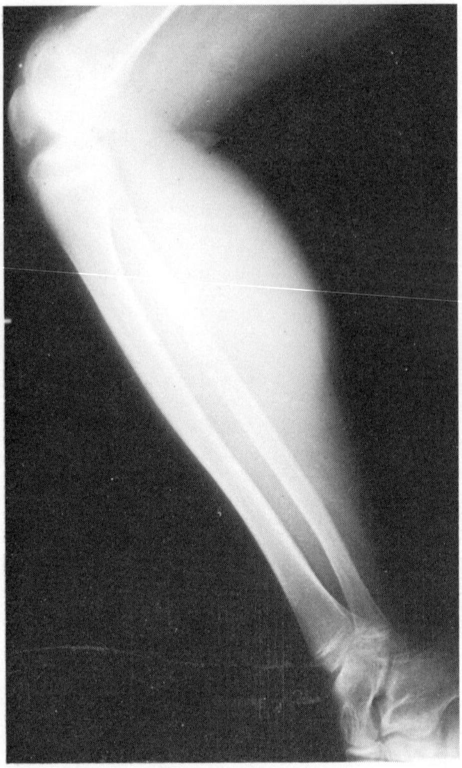

Fig. 23.

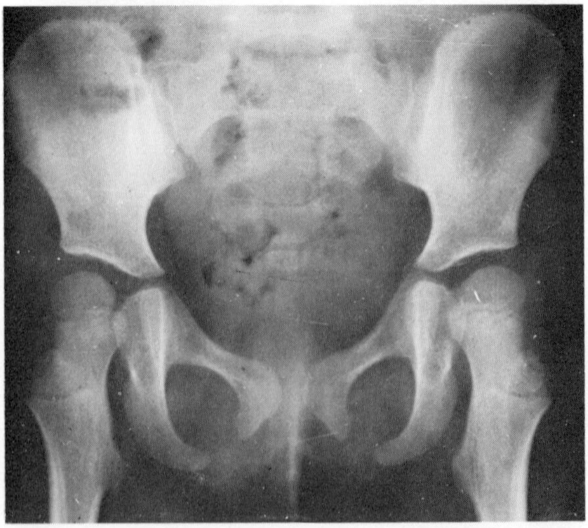

Fig. 24.

BIBLIOGRAPHY

Epstein, B. S. and Abramson, J. L. (1941), 'Roentgenologic Changes in the Bones in Cases of Pseudohypertrophic Muscular Dystrophy,' *Arch. Neurol. Psychiat.*, **46,** 868–876.

Gay, B. B., Jr. and Weems, H. S. (1973), 'Roentgenologic Evaluation of Disorders of Muscle,' *Seminars in Roentgenology*, **VIII,** No. 1.

Lewitan, A. and Nathanson, L. (1955), 'The Roentgen Features of Muscular Dystrophy,' *Amer. J. Roentgenol.*, **73,** No. 2, 226–234.

CHAPTER 8

Problems of Care in Muscular Dystrophy

Respiratory
Infection
Cor Pulmonale
Cardiomyopathy
Fractures
Dental Problems
Pregnancy
Gastrointestinal
Gastric Dilatation
Rectal Prolapse
Fecal Impaction
Obesity
Dystrophia Myotonica
Differential Muscular Weakness
Skin Changes
Speech Problems

In addition to facing specific functional orthopaedic problems secondary to weakness and contracture, muscular dystrophy patients suffer a variety of primary and secondary difficulties requiring clinical understanding and attention.

The protean manifestations of polymyositis are described in detail elsewhere in this text. They include not only inflammatory muscle disease but also skin lesions, neoplasm and collagen-vascular features.

Respiratory

Respiratory infection is an ever present problem in cases of muscular dystrophy. Decrease in respiratory function can lead to cor pulmonale, with right heart failure and cardiomyopathy. Primary cardiomyopathy is noted in well over 50% of patients with Duchenne muscular dystrophy, as well as occurring in the other myopathies.

Fractures

As muscular enfeeblement advances, patients tend to fall more frequently and fractures are common. These can be treated along standard orthopaedic lines because dystrophic bones, although often slender and osteoporotic, heal satisfactorily. In fact, with less muscle power remaining, so that minimal muscle contraction is available to pull against a break, there is, in muscular dystrophy, often less deformity and less pain than normally expected with fractures. Deterioration in muscle strength inevitably follows enforced periods of immobilization, and fractures should be treated ambulatory whenever feasible.

Because of facial muscular weakness and difficulty maintaining head control, malocclusion is frequent, chewing difficult, and dental problems common. Dental hygiene is poor and treatment often difficult. If a general anaesthetic is necessary for dental care, it should always be administered in a hospital.

Several speech defects are associated with muscular dystrophy. Duchenne dystrophics often suffer diminished speed of the diadochokinetic movements of the jaw and tongue, errors of articulation and a thin voice quality characterized by excessive nasality (dystrophic voice). Also, if the tongue is enlarged, the speech may be indistinct. In facioscapulohumeral dystrophy, immobility of the upper lip leads to distortions, substitutions and omissions of labial sounds in all positions.

Pregnancy

In adult forms of muscle disease, pregnancy is usually uneventful although there is sometimes loss of muscle power during the third trimester. The myometrium is not affected in the muscular dystrophies, and therefore, labour is usually normal. However, in dystrophia myotonica, assistance is often required during the second stage of labour.

Gastrointestinal

Acute gastric dilatation has been reported in progressive muscular dystrophy, and smooth muscle involvement (particularly that of the GI tract) has been noted on autopsy in this disease. Rectal prolapse can be seen secondary to sphincter weakness. Fecal impaction is a complication of terminal muscle disease. Obesity is a severe complication in the wheelchair-confined patient with any form of muscular dystrophy.

Dystrophia Myotonica

The full spectrum of clinical involvement in dystrophia myotonica has been covered elsewhere in this book. In addition to progressive weakness and myotonia, this complex multisystem disease includes dysphagia, Pickwickian syndrome (secondary to the CO_2 narcosis of alveolar hypoventilation *and relieved by intermittent positive pressure breathing*), hypogonadism, hypothyroidism, pituitary diabetes, stellate cataract, hyperostosis cranii, cardiac myopathy, temporal baldness, and mental and social deterioration.

Differential Muscular Weakness

The patho-kinetics of progressive muscle disease are essentially the same in distribution and sequence in all the muscular dystrophies. The difference lies in the degree and rapidity of progression of weakness and contracture. For instance, although neck extensors, tibialis posterior and toe flexors are commonly spared in all types, all groups show involvement of lower and middle trapezii. There are, however, some exceptions to this general rule. For example, in Duchenne dystrophy, the anterior neck flexors (particularly sternocleidomastoid) are involved more frequently than in the other myopathies. Hamstring strength is usually preserved in Duchenne dystrophy (lateral hamstrings are spared the longest). In limb-girdle dystrophy, the brachioradialis is commonly strong, whereas in facioscapulohumeral dystrophy, lower pectoralis major is often spared, although tibialis anticus is frequently involved early in the disease.

In all the common dystrophies, the pattern of loss is from proximal to distal. Duchenne and limb-girdle dystrophy are symmetrical in distribution, whereas facioscapulohumeral dystrophy may be asymmetrical. Flexors are usually weaker than extensors in the trunk and neck, whereas extensors are usually weaker than flexors in the hips and shoulders. However, triceps brachii may be stronger than biceps brachii in the Becker's (late appearing, slow evolving) form of Duchenne muscular dystrophy. One of the earliest signs of facioscapulohumeral dystrophy (even in forme fruste cases) can be finger or wrist extensor weakness.

Most major axial or appendicular musculature requires at least 33% anatomical muscle loss before critical weakness becomes obvious clinically. This accounts for the apparent normal function of children with Duchenne muscular dystrophy during the first several years of life. It may also explain the ostensible improvement of such patients from age five to seven years because in these cases, the processes of normal development, utilizing residual muscle strength, outstrip the progress of their disease.

Skin Changes

There is some evidence that in addition to muscle involvement Duchenne dystrophy causes primary and secondary changes in the collagen vascular system. A subcutaneous reticular vascular pattern (livedo reticularis), accentuated by exercise, is seen in these patients. Another skin condition (erythema ab igne) is also frequent in Duchenne muscular dystrophics, as is seborrheic dermatitis. In addition, non-specific changes in subcutaneous fat have been reported.

Although some hearing loss has been reported in patients with facio-scapulohumeral dystrophy, the hearing acuity of children with Duchenne muscular dystrophy is essentially normal in spite of an increased response latency.

Speech Problems

Speech problems are often noted in the muscular dystrophies. In facioscapulohumeral disease, where weakness begins in the facial musculature, patients may have difficulty with speech, characterized by misarticulated sounds and substitutions, omissions and distortions of the labial sounds (P, B, M, W) in all positions in words. This is due to weakness of the obicularis oris muscle. The speech characteristics of advanced Duchenne dystrophy include diminished diadochokinetic rates of tongue and jaw movements, moderate to severe articular disorders (if the tongue is hypertrophied, indistinct speech may be apparent), 'dystrophic voice', a thin vocal quality with excessive nasality, and an impairment in laryngeal control, manifested by an inability to cough, clear the throat, or sustain phonation. In addition, vocal intensity is lower than average. In ocular muscular dystrophy (a rare disease) the facial and

Chart 6. Speech Therapy Exercises

Lip Exercises

1. Alternate puckering and smiling, simultaneously producing *oo-ee*. Practice in front of a mirror.
2. Pucker lips and fill cheeks with air. Keeping lips tightly pursed, depress inflated cheeks with fingertips and strive to keep air within the oral cavity. Do not allow any air to escape through the puckered lips, or to be swallowed.
3. Insert a lifesaver or button (of varying sizes) strung on dental floss between closed teeth and compressed lips. Individual should strive to retain the lifesaver or button behind the tightly puckered lips while the therapist pulls on the dental floss, gradually increasing the resistance. This is particularly good in maintaining the strength of the orbicularis oris.
4. Tucking the lips in until none of the red border can be seen.
5. Puckering the lips, and moving the pursed lips from side to side as far as they will go.
6. Compressing and releasing the lips rapidly, with the sounds *mee . . . mee . . . mee*, then changing to *pah . . . pah . . . pah*, *poh . . . poh . . . poh*, *bee . . . bee . . . bee*, and *wah . . . wah . . . wah*.

Tongue Exercises

1. Mrs Tongue Story or Circus Acts (done in front of mirror).
2. Lingual lateralization.

Palatal Exercises

1. Blowing exercises are effective in maintaining the function of the palatal muscles: Blowing bubbles in water through a straw, balloons, toy horns, whistles, a ping-pong ball or a feather across a table, and pinwheels. Also, blowing a toy boat in a pan of water or in the bathtub, using the sound *oo* (as in boot).
2. Repeating syllables: *Ung-gah*, *ung-gah*, *ung-gah*, with the mouth open and no movement of the jaws.
3. Letting the child feel the difference between nasal and mouth sounds by placing his fingers on the bridge of your nose. Sing *m-m-m-m*, then sing *ah-ah*.
4. Emphasizing the fact that only m, n, and ng come through the nose by having the child feel the bridge of his nose as he pretends to be a humming top and says *m-m-m*, then changes to *ah* . . ..
5. Practicing word lists for rapid adjustment from nasalized to non-nasalized sounds (ex. sambo, ramble, amber, tamper, lamp).

oropharyngeal muscles are commonly involved, leading to both dysphonia and dysphagia. In dystrophia myotonica, particularly the childhood form, speech is nasal and often indistinct. This may be due to the slow myotonic relaxation of tongue muscles following the strong voluntary contraction which is pathognomonic of this form of dystrophy. Oropharyngeal weakness affects speech in many cases, and dysphagia is sometimes a serious problem. A sustained downwards displacement of the soft palate during speaking or swallowing causing nasality has been attributed to myotonia of the tensor veli palatini.

Although it has been suggested that in the rapidly progressing forms of muscular dystrophy, attempts at speech therapy would be futile, most speech therapists feel that in the more slowly progressive types such treatment may be beneficial as well as moral-building. Therefore, speech therapy has been utilized to maintain articulation skills and/or to compensate for indistinctness due to impaired lip, tongue and soft palate movements.

Chart 6 illustrates some therapy techniques that may be useful in maintaining strength and range of movement of the lips, tongue and soft palate.

Thus, we see that total care of the dystrophic patient covers a variety of systems, requiring an understanding of the many facets of these diseases and the application of a variety of diagnostic and therapeutic skills.

BIBLIOGRAPHY

Abramson, A. S. (1958). *An Approach to the Rehabilitation of Children with Muscular Dystrophy*. Muscular Dystrophy Associations of America, Incorporated, Scientific Department. MDA Inc. Pub. No. 0, 101.

Allen, Nell R. (1973), 'Hearing Acuity in Patients with Muscular Dystrophy,' *Develop. Med. Child Neurol.* **15,** 500–505.

Huvos, A. G. and Pruzanski, W. (1967), 'Smooth Muscle Involvement in Primary Muscle Disease. I. Myotonic Dystrophy,' *Arch. Path.*, **83,** 229–233.

Huvos, A. G. and Pruzanski, W. (1967), 'Smooth Muscle Involvement in Primary Muscle Disease. II. Progressive Muscular Dystrophy,' *Arch. Path.*, **83,** 234–240.

Robin, G. C. and Falewski, G. DeL. (1963), 'Acute Gastric Dilatation in Progressive Muscular Dystrophy,' *Lancet* (Original Articles), **ii,** 171–172.

Mullendore, J. M. and Stoudt, R. J., Jr. (1961), Speech Patterns of Muscular Dystrophic Individuals,' *J. Speech Hear. Dis.*, **26,** No. 3, 252–257.

Voda, Jerrilyn A., CCC-SP, Director, Department of Speech Pathology, London Memorial Hospital, Chicago, Illinois. Personal Communication.

CHAPTER 9

Cardiomyopathy

Cardiomyopathy is a complication of all forms of muscular dystrophy. It is very common in Duchenne dystrophy. It may be seen in limb-girdle dystrophy. It also frequently occurs in dystrophia myotonica, and although uncommon in facioscapulohumeral dystrophy, it has been found. Nonspecific T-wave changes can be seen in polymyositis, but clinical signs of cardiac disease rarely develop.

Symptoms

Although most patients with Duchenne muscular dystrophy die of inanition and pulmonary infection, dystrophic cardiomyopathy is also an important cause of death. Cardiac disease may be simulated, obscured or aggravated by weakness of the chest bellows and diaphragm, or deformity of the thorax and recurrent lower respiratory infection. Dyspnea, fatigue, and tachycardia are provoked by muscular effort. Sudden episodes of palpitation, diaphoresis, emesis, and abdominal pain may occur. However, the patient may not show clinical evidence of heart disease even though myocardial dystrophy is noted on the electrocardiogram. Restricted activity maintains a precarious clinical status quo. Rapidly progressive preterminal heart failure often occurs after years of such clinical stability. Thoracic deformity and an elevated diaphragm make physical and X-ray examination of the heart difficult. Nonetheless, the following auscultatory pathology may be found:

1. Increased incidence of third and fourth heart sounds (quadruple rhythm).
2. Occasionally a murmur of mitral regurgitation secondary to dystrophic involvement of a papillary muscle or adjacent myocardium may disappear with treatment and may be confused with the murmur of tricuspid regurgitation in patients with right heart involvement or strain.
3. Dysrhythmias:
    a. labile sinus tachycardia
    b. premature beats (atrial or ventricular)
    c. atrial flutter
    d. paroxysmal ventricular tachycardia.

Enzyme quantification has sometimes been helpful in detecting myocardial dystrophy. The lactic dehydrogenase isozyme profile of dystrophic skeletal muscle resembles that of cardiac muscle, and meaningful distinction cannot be made. However, CPK isozymes have been useful in detecting heart muscle involvement in Duchenne dystrophy.

EKG Changes

Vectorcardiography can often detect otherwise obscure pathology, but this technique is not available to the average practitioner. However, cardiomyopathy, with or without cardiac insufficiency, can be suspected because of certain typical patterns seen on a standard 12-lead scalar electrocardiogram (Fig. 25). These include:

1. Tall right precordial R waves with increased R/S ratios (V_1 and V_{3R}) which may progress to the development of incomplete right bundle branch block with eventual disappearance of the tall R wave.
2. Deep limb lead and lateral precordial Q waves (specifically seen in sex-linked Duchenne dystrophy).
3. Deep Q waves co-existing with an altered shape of the right precordial R waves (RSR or polyphasic R waves).
4. At a later stage diffuse myocardial damage may appear, manifested by inverted T waves, ST segment deviation, and abnormal Q waves.

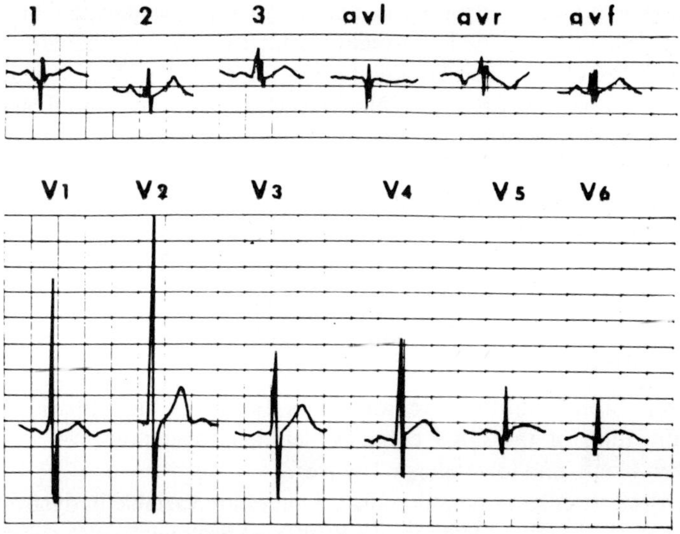

Fig. 25. Some typical EKG findings in cardiomyopathy. (14-year-old boy with Duchenne muscular dystrophy.)
Note: 1. Narrow but deep Q waves in leads 1, avl, V_5 and V_6.
2. RSR pattern in avr.
3. Dominant (R) waves in V_1 and V_2.
(Modified from *Disorders of Voluntary Muscle*, 3rd Edn. (1974) by courtesy of J. N. Walton, M.D. (Ed.) and Churchill Livingstone.)

As discussed in the section on the carrier state, creatine phosphokinase quantification has been used to identify female carriers of Duchenne muscular dystrophy. Electrocardiograms which are distinctive of Duchenne muscular dystrophy have also been found in some female carriers whose only other manifestation of myopathic disease is an elevated CPK.

Limb-girdle dystrophy shows cardiac involvement uncommonly, but when present, it expresses itself as:

1. Disturbances in rhythm or conduction (QRS prolongation, first-degree heart block, right ventricular conduction defects, atrial flutter).
2. Abnormal Q waves and minor T wave alterations.
3. Third and fourth heart sounds (quadruple rhythm).
4. Overt heart failure.

In this form of dystrophy, symptoms such as dyspnea, cough, and lower respiratory infection usually result from an inadequate chest bellows rather than cardiac failure. On the other hand, dyspnea and cough in a patient with Duchenne muscular dystrophy should be considered of cardiac origin until proven otherwise.

Cardiac involvement is rare in facioscapulohumeral dystrophy although occasional examples of mild occult cardiac disease occur.

The manifestations of cardiomyopathy in dystrophia myotonica consist of:

1. Asymptomatic EKG abnormalities.
2. Overt rhythm and conduction disturbances.
3. Heart failure.

EKG abnormalities include sinus bradycardia, slurring and prolongation of the QRS complex (left axis deviation), left bundle branch block, and low voltage T waves.

Atrioventricular conduction disturbances are variable in dystrophia myotonica. Anything from mild PR interval prolongation to complete atrioventricular block has been seen. Disturbances of rhythm consist chiefly of atrial flutter or fibrillation. Sometimes cardiac enlargement and heart failure may accompany dystrophia myotonica. Usually, systemic myotonia is clinically present long before cardiomyopathy becomes overt. Occasionally, cardiac symptoms dominate the clinical picture, and cardiac involvement is sometimes responsible for sudden death. Antimyotonic medication should be cautiously prescribed where cardiomyopathy is present as Quinine, Dilantin and procaine amide all affect the myocardium.

Finally, patients with advanced myopathy, particularly those wheelchair confined, sometimes compensate for severe lumbar lordosis through flattening their normal thoracic kyphosis. A 'straight back syndrome' can occur which may mimic organic heart disease by causing systolic murmur (owing to impingement or distortion of great vessels) and cardiac compression (secondary to decrease in AP chest diameter). This results in pseudocardiomegaly and/or an abnormal electrocardiogram. Recognition of this 'pseudoheart disease' can avoid iatrogenic cardiac disease with consequent overtreatment.

Pathology

The essential pathologic changes in cardiomyopathy consist of cardiac muscle atrophy, with replacement of fibres by collagenous connective tissue, blending with the sacroplasm of adjacent cardiac muscle fibres (Fig. 26). Fibroplastic proliferation is not seen, and the cellular content of the connective tissue probably represents surviving cardiac nuclei. Fat replacement (as noted in the skeletal muscle of progressive muscular dystrophy) is not a feature of the dystrophic myocardial process. EKG patterns may reflect either dystrophic lesions in the myocardium, or less likely, abnormal persistence of the EKG of early childhood.

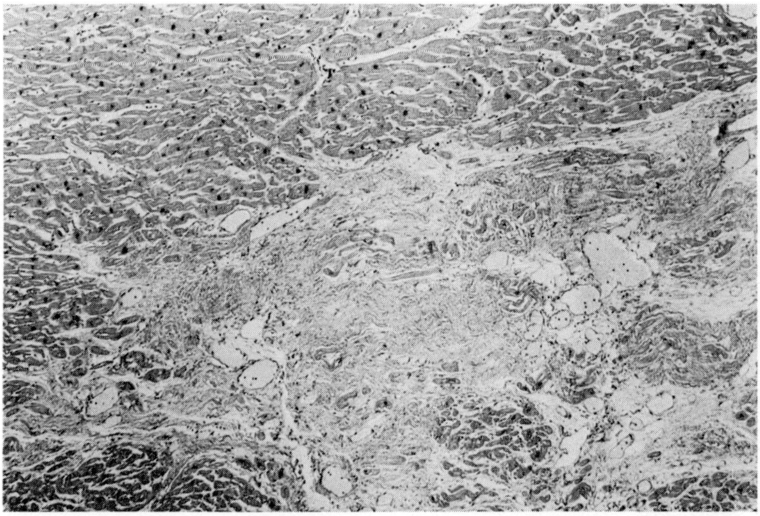

Fig. 26. Histopathologic changes in cardiopathy.

When labile sinus tachycardia occurs, it is usually due to disease of the nodal arteries. The role played by the autonomic nervous system is not known. Chronic congestive heart failure, though rare, has been found. In children who have the slow (Becker's) form of Duchenne's dystrophy, serious dystrophic cardiomyopathy may be present, and these patients stand a significant risk of sudden cardiac death.

BIBLIOGRAPHY

Datey, K. K., Deshmukh, M. M., Engineer, S. D. and Dalvi, C. P. (1964), 'Straight Back Syndrome,' *Brit. Heart J.*, **26,** 614–619.

DeLeon, A. C., Jr., Perloff, J. K., Twigg, H. and Majd, M. (1965), 'The Straight Back Syndrome. Clinical Cardiovascular Manifestations,' *Circulation*, **32,** 193–203.

Diaz, F. V., Pelous, A. N., Valdes, F. G., Grande, F. G. G. and Granados, A. (1962), 'Pectus Exavatum. Hemodynamic and Electrocardiographic Considerations (Case Reports),' *Amer. J. Cardiol.*, **10,** 272–277.

Gooch, A. S., Maranhao, V., Goldberg, H. and Mills, B. (1967), 'The Straight Thoracic Spine in Cardiac Diagnosis,' *Amer. Heart J.*, **74,** No. 5, 595–602.

Norris Jr., F. H., Moss, A. J. and Yu, Paul, N. (1966), 'On the Possibility that a Type of Human Muscular Dystrophy Commences in Myocardium,' *Ann. N.Y. Acad. Sci.*, **138,** Article 1, 342–354.

Perloff, J. K. (1971), 'Cardiomyopathy Associated with Heredofamilial Neuromyopathic Diseases,' *Modern Concepts of Cardiovascular Diseases*, **XL,** No. 5, 23–26.

Rawlings, M. S. (1960), 'The "Straight Back" Sydrome. A new Cause of Pseudoheart Disease,' *Amer. J. Cardiol.*, **5,** 333–338.

Reusch, C. S. (1961), 'Hemodynamic Studies in Pectus Excavatum,' *Circulation*, **24,** 1143–1150.

Siegel, I. M. (1972), 'Cardiomyopathy: Presenting Symptom of Progressive Muscular Dystrophy,' *J. Amer. med. Ass.*, **222,** No. 8 (Letters), 1060.

Siegel, J. S. and Schecter, E. (1967), 'The Straight Back Syndrome. Another Cause of Innocent Systolic Murmurs,' *Amer. J. Med.*, **42,** 309–313.

Slucka, Cecylia, (1968), 'The Electrocardiogram in Duchenne Progressive Muscular Dystrophy,' *Circulation*, **38,** 933–940.

Teplick, G. J. and Drake, E. H. (1946), 'The Roentgen and Cardiac Manifestations of Funnel Chest,' *Amer. J. Roentgenol.*, **56,** No. 6, 721–735.

Walton, J. N. (Ed.) (1974), *Disorders of Voluntary Muscles*, 3rd edition. London: J. & A. Churchill, Ltd.

CHAPTER 10

Pulmonary Complications

Pneumonia

Pneumonia secondary to inanition, decreased pulmonary function, and poor respiratory toilet with aspiration is a frequent problem in advanced cases of muscular dystrophy, and the most common cause of death. Occurrence of sudden demise in patients with dystrophic myocardial involvement may be due to acute congestive heart failure following a sudden demand, secondary to pneumonitis, on a limited cardiac reserve. This is, no doubt, an important contributory cause of death where the primary factor is pneumonia. This mechanism may also play a role in the sudden death which sometimes follows attacks of abdominal pain, emesis, and diarrhoea. This common complication in bed-ridden patients leads to dehydration and electrolyte imbalance. Such a state is poorly tolerated by the dystrophic myocardium, and sudden death can result.

The pneumonias that are typically encountered in muscular dystrophy are hypostatic, involving the left lower, right lower, and right middle lobes of the lungs. Weakness of swallowing compounds the infection by increasing the danger of aspiration. Debility of the oropharynx often prevents a patient from learning to breathe with his pharynx ('frog' breathing). Cough is poor because these patients lack the respiratory capacity and expiratory reserve volume with which to exert sufficient force to cough effectively. Antihistamine decongestants should not be prescribed as they increase mucous inspissation and further irritate the respiratory passages.

Aspiration pneumonia has also been reported as a common cause of death in patients with dystrophia myotonica. In addition to decreased vital capacity, suggesting a weakened chest bellows and restrictive ventilatory defect without obstruction, these patients commonly suffer pulmonary infections because of an inability of the esophagus to adequately empty, permitting nocturnal aspiration and further pulmonary embarrassment.

Treatment

Cardiomyopathy in muscular dystrophy is managed with the same techniques and agents as in non-dystrophic patients. Cardiac glycosides,* diuretics, etc. are used. Pneumonia is vigorously treated with fluids, antipyretics, ventilatory therapy and early antimicrobial treatment appropriate to the causative agent. In those patients with dystrophia myotonica demonstrating decrease of esophageal motility, bed elevation at night is recommended to prevent possible aspiration pneumonitis. Youngsters with Duchenne dystrophy are encouraged in deep breathing (blow bottles, balloon blowing) and, where possible, induced to play wind instruments.

In all patients, as pulmonary function diminishes, diaphragmatic (and even pharyngeal) breathing techniques are taught and vigorously practiced (Chart 7). 'Range of motion' of the chest must be maintained. Proper humidification is provided at home to avoid upper respiratory infections (particularly bronchitis) which may progress to more serious pulmonary disease. Respiratory vaccines are administered to increase resistance, smoking is interdict. A programme of postural drainage and chest therapy (Chart 8) becomes part of the daily routine (Fig. 27). A foot-operated suction apparatus for home use may be helpful in removing secretions from the posterior pharynx. A portable intermittent positive pressure breathing apparatus, activated by a small pressure tank or mechanical pump can maintain maximal available

* The myopathic heart is usually sensitive to even small doses of digitalis.

Chart 7. Technique of Diaphragmatic Breathing

To use the diaphragm effectively, the abdomen must rise with inspiration and fall with expiration. With the therapist's hands placed over the lower ribs, the patient is instructed to push the therapist's hands out with inspiration and allow them to move inward with expiration.

With the patient in a supine position, the therapist places a hand or weight on the upper abdomen. Emphasis is placed on the proper sequence of diaphragmatic breathing. On inspiration, the abdomen rises first, next the lower ribs push out, finally the chest rises.

All diaphragmatic breathing exercises are done with the shoulders relaxed. Patients are encouraged to relax and taught to breathe with the diaphragm, keeping the upper chest still.

In the seated position, patients are instructed to sit straight with the arms abducted and on inspiration expand the chest as much as possible. On expiration the patient bends forward at the waist, bringing his arms down and across his chest, and forces a maximal expiration.

Following are some specific instructions given to children on this programme:

1. Lie on the floor on your back. Now bend your knees, keeping your feet flat on the floor. Hold your hands over your abdomen. Now breathe in through your nose. Your abdomen should go out like a balloon. Try to relax your upper chest and shoulders. Do this ten times slowly.
2. Breathe again like above, only this time blow the air out through your pursed lips. Close your lips as though you were trying to whistle. Pulling the air in through your nose, your abdomen goes up. Blowing the air out through your lips, your abdomen goes down.
3. Count to yourself as you practice this way of breathing. Count to two as you breathe in through your nose. Count to four slowly as you blow out through your pursed lips. Blowing out is the most important. Use your hands on your abdomen to help press all the air out. Do this ten times slowly.
4. Put a book on your abdomen. See if you can make the book rise up as you take in air and make your abdomen round. Your abdomen should get flat again as you blow all the air out. While you are doing this, try to relax your chest and shoulders.
5. Sit up straight in a chair. Put a candle in front of you on a table, with the flame at the level of your mouth. Now hold your hands against your abdomen. Breathe in some air and let your abdomen push out against your hands. Now, blow out gently towards the flame through your pursed lips. See if you can bend the flame. As you blow, press gently on your abdomen. Move the candle away a little bit each day until it is two feet away. Can you still bend the flame?
6. Sit in a chair and put a ping-pong ball in front of you on a table. Blow out gently through your pursed lips towards the ball. Mark how far it goes. See if you can blow it a little farther the next time.

Chart 8. Chest Therapy Programme

The following manoeuvres are helpful in mobilizing respiratory secretions. They are most effective when combined with aerosol and IPPB therapy.

1. **Postural drainage.** The body is placed in various positions to promote drainage of specific segments of the lung. When those bronchi draining a lung segment are perpendicular, gravity will assist the flow of secretions.

   A. Upper lobes, anterior segments both lungs: Semi-Fowler's position, sitting at 45° angle.
   B. Lingular and lateral segments, left lower lobe: Right side lying $\frac{1}{4}$ turn from supine, foot of bed elevated 12–14 inches.
   C. Posterior segments, left lower lobe: Right side lying $\frac{1}{4}$ turn from prone, foot of bed elevated.
   D. Anterior segments, both lower lobes: Supine—foot of bed elevated.
   E. Posterior segments, right lower lobe: Left side lying $\frac{1}{4}$ turn from prone, foot of bed elevated.
   F. Middle lobe, right lung: Left side lying $\frac{1}{4}$ turn from supine, foot of bed elevated.

2. **Chest percussion.** In this manoeuvre, the chest is 'clapped' with cupped hands to loosen secretions adhering to broncheolar walls.
3. **Chest vibration and compression.** The flattened palms of the hands are placed on the chest wall. The arms and hands are vibrated while compressing the chest. This assists exhalation and encourages coughing.

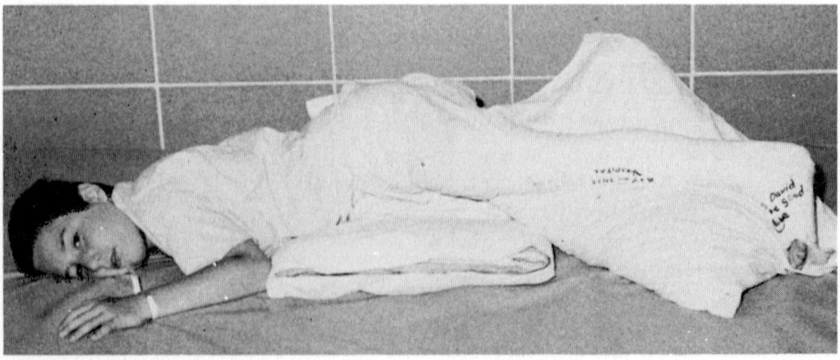

Fig. 27. Position for postural drainage.

respiratory function and, at least, delay pulmonary complication as long as feasible.

Chronic Alveolar Hypoventilation

Chronic alveolar hypoventilation has been reported in all the major forms of muscular dystrophy. Inadequate gaseous exchange across the lungs leads to hypoxemia, retention of carbon dioxide, and respiratory acidosis. Clinical symptoms include somnolence or confusion, sometimes with headache, blurred vision, and diplopia. There may be various degrees of organic mental disorder with coma, asterixis (and other movement disorders), papilledema, irregular respiration, cyanosis, and manifestations of right heart failure. Clinical findings are associated with increased arterial carbon dioxide tension. Under these circumstances, respiratory control is modulated primarily by the action of lowered arterial oxygen tension on the carotid receptors. As in other chronic respiratory conditions, inhaling pure oxygen may have a deleterious effect.

Pickwickian Syndrome

Pickwickian syndrome is sometimes seen (particularly in dystrophia myotonica), and other related findings include insomnia, headaches, nightmares, apprehension and hyperhidrosis. Intermittent positive pressure respiration, combined with weight reduction and diuretics, is the treatment of choice in such patients.

In the later stages of muscular dystrophy there is a significant loss of ventilation with ineffective cough, and minor respiratory infections can be devastating. Fear and fatique contribute to this peripheral respiratory failure. Objective signs include secondary polycythemia, elevated heart rate, increase in CO_2 combining power, reduced vital capacity, decreased cough force, reduced chest expansion and a change in breathing pattern (laboured hyperpnea). A hand resuscitator (Emerson type) is useful at home to encourage hyperventilation and decrease cough. A portable home IPPB thereapy unit is also advised* (Fig. 28). Later, a mechanical respirator may be necessary. If breathing becomes seriously laboured, particularly if cough force is poor or cough reflex absent and vital capacity is less than 50% expected value, tracheostomy is required to assist ventilation and relieve breathing fatique.

* Retec, Model NC-30, fluid cycling valve and nebulizer, Everest and Jennings, Inc., Los Angeles, California.

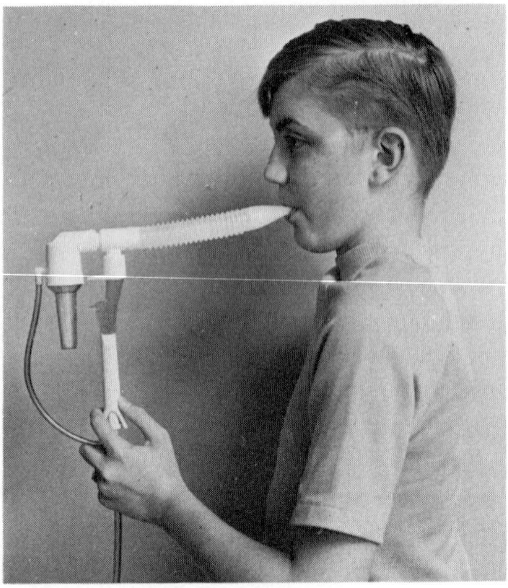

Fig. 28. Portable intermittent positive pressure breathing apparatus (Retec NC-30, Everest and Jennings, Inc., Los Angeles, Calif.) in use.

Thus, the three major goals in respiratory care are:

1. The maintenance of respiratory homeostasis, through
2. training in the use of the various types of respiratory aids, therefore
3. enabling the patient to lead as active and as comfortable a life as possible within the limits imposed by his evolving respiratory problems.

BIBLIOGRAPHY

Aberion, Graciela, Alba, A., Lee, M. H. M. and Solomon, M. (1973), 'Pulmonary Care of Duchenne Type of Muscular Dystrophy,' *N. Y. St. J. Med.*, **73,** pp. 1206—1207.

Adams, Marjorie A. and Chandler, Lynette S. (1974), 'Effects of Physical Therapy Program on Vital Capacity of Patients with Muscular Dystrophy,' *Phys. Ther.*, **54,** No. 5, 494–496.

Adkins, Hazel V. (1968), 'Improvement of Breathing Ability in Children with Respiratory Muscle Paralysis,' *Phys. Ther.*, **48,** No. 6, 577–581.

Buchsbaum, H. D., Martin, W. A., Turino, G. M. and Rowland, L. P. (1968), 'Chronic Alveolar Hypoventilation Due to Muscular Dystrophy,' *Neurol.*, **18,** No. 4, 319–327.

Burke, S. S., Grove, N. M., Houser, Carolyn R. and Johnson, Donna M. (1971), 'Respiratory Aspects of Pseudo-hypertrophic Muscular Dystrophy,' *Amer. J. Dis. Child.*, **121,** 230–234.

Dail, C. W. (1965), 'Respiratory Aspects of Rehabilitation in Neuromuscular Conditions,' *Arch. phys. Med. Rehab.*, **46,** 655–675.

Garrett, J. M., DuBose, T. J., Jr., Jackson, J. E. and Norman, J. R. (1969), 'Esophageal and Pulmonary Disturbances in Myotonica Dystrophica,' *Arch. intern. Med.*, **123,** 26–32.

Greenberg, M. and Edmonds, J. (1974), 'Chronic Respiratory Problems in Neuromyopathic Disorders—Their Nature and Management,' *Pediat. Clin. N. Amer.*, **21,** No. 4, 927–934.

Houser, Carolyn R. and Johnson, Donna M. (1971), 'Breathing Exercises for Children with Pseudohypertrophic Muscular Dystrophy,' *Phys. Ther.*, **51,** No. 7, 751–759.

Inkley, S. R., Oldenburg, F. C. and Vignos, P. J. (1974), 'Pulmonary Function in Duchenne Muscular Dystrophy Related to Stage of Disease,' *Amer. J. Med.*, **56,** 297–306.

McCormack, W. M. and Spalter, H. D. (1966), 'Muscular Dystrophy, Alveolar Hypoventilation and Papilledema,' *J. Amer. med. Ass.*, **197,** 957.

Neustadt, J. E., Levy, R. C. and Spiegel, I. J. (1964), 'Carbon Dioxide Narcosis in Association with Muscular Dystrophy,' *J. Amer. med Ass.*, **187,** 616.

Sackner, M. A. (1975), 'Diaphragmatic Breathing Exercises: Therapy in Chronic Obstructive Pulmonary Disease,' *J. Amer. med. Ass.*, **231,** No. 3, 295–296.

Saheki, B., Fukuyama, K., Miyoshi, M. Tani, J. and Koshiyama, K. (1967), 'The Studies on the Pulmonary Function of the Patients of Progressive Muscular Dystrophy,' *Iryo*, **21,** No. 7, 23–30.

Siegel, I. M. (1975), 'Pulmonary Problems in Duchenne Muscular Dystrophy: Diagnosis, Prophylaxis, and Treatment,' *Phys. Ther.*, **55,** No. 2, 160–162.

CHAPTER 11

Psychological and Social Problems

Importance

Muscular dystrophy is a crippling, progressive, and fatal disease. Most parents and many patients know this. However, they should also be made aware of the intensive research being conducted to discover the cause and cure of the dystrophies. Such discoveries are real possibilities. Therefore, the patient must be prepared for the future. Attention to the social and psychological factors relevant to these diseases may make the difference between relative future well being and inactivity and unhappiness.

Honest Expectations

A life space must be provided for such patients, so that they may live productively and as normally as possible while realistically recognizing the specific limitations imposed by their disease. Honest expectations must be set for these children, as is the case with any crippling disease. At the same time, one should avoid overprotection, allowing the child to accomplish by his own efforts those tasks which win for him the approbation of his environment. Such overprotection, rather than helping, leads inevitably to isolation and dependency. Therefore, as a general rule, such children should be encouraged to attend an ordinary school as long as feasible, and vocational training where appropriate should be geared toward a career enabling the child to undertake an occupation within the limits of his disability.

There are no distinct psychopathologic entities exclusive to muscular dystrophy, and severe emotional illness is no more common than in a normal population. In fact, there is a surprising absence of psychiatric problems among even the most severely physically incapacitated children. However, because progressive disability is so devastatingly overwhelming, any defence should be encouraged if it is not harmful.

The association of muscular dystrophy and lowered intelligence quotient has been documented. Upwards of 25% of such patients (most frequently Duchenne dystrophics) show intellectual deficits. There is some suggestion of an early nonprogressive intellectual impairment of verbal intelligence as well as a greater than normal incidence of diffuse EEG abnormalities. Although these findings suggest the possibility of an organic etiology for retardation in muscular dystrophy, they may also reflect depressed functioning secondary to the psychological, social and educational impositions of the disease which prevent patients from realizing their intellectual potential. Where mental retardation is found, a sibling with the disease will usually (concordantly) also show such a deficit.

Most patients with muscular dystrophy are emotionally dependent and lack frustration tolerance. They tend toward social and emotional withdrawal and, failing to develop dominant modes of conscious attitudes, favour emotional seesawing and impulsive responses. Also, as would be expected, such children tend to deal, even more than the normal, in fantasy.

The family with a handicapped child need not necessarily be a handicapped family. In considering the psychological aspects of chronic illness, we should realize that any illness in a child represents a family crisis. Just how this crisis is resolved depends upon the pre-existing strength of the family unit. It requires great strength, stability, and support to sustain a muscular dystrophic child in a family.

Factors in Management

Factors to be considered in the management of the dystrophic child and his family include:

1. The child's personality and needs.
2. The child's stage of emotional development and its vulnerabilities.
3. The child's perception of his illness and its management.
4. The nature of the dystrophy in itself and its potential effects on the child and his family.
5. The nature of management procedure and the potential for support of the child from his family and physician.

Child's Adjustment

The adjustment of a child with muscular dystrophy will be effected by a number of things, including:

1. The need for parental separation at any time during disease (children who are separated for long periods of time from parents show adverse reactions, characterized by a stage of protest, followed by a stage of despair which terminates in a final stage of detachment or denial).
2. Restriction, including sensory impairment and isolation. When normal avenues of play are restricted, a child may withdraw into excessive fantasy as a means of coping.
3. Dependency and lack of consistency.
4. Pain and deformity. This includes the threat of surgery and fears of being defective and hence an inadequate person.
5. The threat of death (it is not usually until age 9 or 10 that a child fully understands death as being both inevitable and irrevocable).
6. Medication. Prolonged, regular use of drugs may be regarded as an imposition by authority figures.
7. Absence from school.

Family's Response

Familial reaction to the diagnosis of a severe, chronic and crippling illness places a great deal of stress on the family unit. The following factors influence the family's response to this stress.

1. The severity of the illness including the prognosis and the availability of an effective treatment.
2. Whether or not the disease is congenital.
3. The age of onset of the disease and of the diagnosis.

4. The presence of a pre-existing emotional disturbance within the family.
5. The nature and effects of the illness itself.
6. The effects of a programme of home management and restrictions on family life.
7. The presence or absence of affected siblings.
8. Repeated hospitalizations and surgical procedures.
9. The cost of the illness, if privately treated.

Specific parental emotional reactions to the diagnosis of muscular dystrophy include denial, anxiety, feelings of guilt, depression, resentment (and rejection), and reactions of shame, embarrassment, or sheer exhaustion. Sibling reactions are also more or less characterized by the same, or similar, emotional states.

Whatever the physician's reaction is, he should realize that, 'what the family needs is empathy, not sympathy; detachment rather than avoidance'.

Management of Family

Management of the family with a muscular dystrophic child or children is based on a recognition that such a situation will have major implications on the life of that family. The diagnosis of this illness can easily precipitate a state of familial crisis, and the family's past history of adjustment may give clues to the nature of potential difficulties.

The physician must recognize that what the family hear and understand may differ considerably from what they have been told. In general, people can assimilate only what they are prepared for emotionally. One important reason for maintaining regular visits with the family is to clarify what they have heard regarding diagnosis, prognosis and management, and to supervise their day to day coping with management problems, both physical and emotional. At the same time, the physician must facilitate the ventilation of anxiety on the part of both the dystrophic child, his parents, and normal siblings. In this light, group therapy is useful in the counselling and assisting of parents of children with muscular dystrophy. Participants benefit from these meetings by developing insight and increasing communication through experience sharing. Liaison should also be maintained with the child's school, as peer relationships are extremely important in his day-to-day life.

Physicians should realize that they are frequently the objects of hostility which is not personally directed. Rather, it is a displacement of of both the patient's and his parents' resentment toward the fact of the child's illness and a reaction against the one who is confronting them with painful realities they would rather not hear. Physicians who respond with hostility or withdrawal to these projected feelings will lose the valuable opportunity of providing needed services at this time of great stress.

Parental Problems

It has been said that in the treatment of muscular dystrophy the family is the patient. Parents of dystrophic children are faced with serious problems of adjustment. Feelings of guilt, leading to penance and a life of servitude to the child, may contribute to the vicious cycle of anger, guilt, self-pity and ultimate rejection, both of self and the patient. Such feelings are more prevalent in the mother, particularly in the sex-linked form of the disease. Fathers, on the other hand, because their work routines are less disrupted by the presence of a seriously ill home-bound child, and because they may feel less responsible in the production of a sex-linked mutation, seem to bear less primary guilt, but frequently more anger and self-pity.

Demands upon the mother's time and strength are severe. Not always tactful neighbours and strangers provoke self-consciousness and shame. Normal siblings are neglected, and, indeed, part of a counsellor's job is to help parents realize the limitations and prospects of the dystrophic child in his home situation and to aid siblings who have to compete with the sick child for parental attention.

Also, anxiety over the hereditary implications of these diseases disturbs parents and siblings alike. Thus, early discovery of carriers and appropriate genetic counselling are necessary.

Counselling

It is the responsibility of the treating physician to offer intelligent and empathetic advice, and to correlate definitive therapy with an ongoing programme of understanding and patient counsel during the early (diagnostic) phase of treatment. Information should be available to parents on demand. The physician must take particular care to see that no credibility gap occurs and that there is no delay in the diagnosis. One ought to be aware of usual parent reactions, including a period of 'mourning', followed by a slow period of 'adaptation'.

Many parents shocked by a diagnosis of muscular dystrophy will panic and spend useless time, funds, and energy seeking a condition with a better prognosis. The doctor should discuss 'shopping' with all parents. They should be encouraged to seek a reputable second opinion, but also advised to return to the primary physician. The hereditary implications of the disease can be briefly discussed during an early interview.

Finally, available treatment should be outlined and parents encouraged that research is being conducted in the search for the cause and cure of the disease. Mostly, one must be prepared emotionally and time-wise to listen as anxious parents unburden themselves.

During long-term follow-up such matters as sibling responsibility *vis-à-vis* the dystrophic child can be discussed. Parents are asked how the family handles problems in the home. They are instructed in how to listen well, how to 'tune in' to their child's problems, and how to 'read between the lines'.

Some of these children's more common worries, including their concern over the trouble they might be causing, are discussed. Indeed, the judicious use of motorized lifts and other aids to daily living may go far in alleviating such concern. Parents should be instructed in the usual dynamics of this situation (e.g. guilt causing overprotectiveness). They need to be taught to use their intuition and told that, even if they have no solution, just indicating that they recognize the problem can go a long way toward solving it.

If and when patients inquire about their disease, including its fatal aspect, they must be given answers commensurate with their understanding which are realistic, yet hopeful. It is important to recognize exactly what the child is asking and respond to this specific request for information, and not to one's own anxieties and fantasies.

One of the critical points in the psychological course of muscular dystrophy occurs when a child can no longer attend school and becomes homebound. At this point, parents must face the ultimate painful recognition of the severity of their child's condition. Also, the mother is now occupied with the patient all day long. A father will often feel guilt in relation to the mother who is so beset by the every day physical and psychological problems of their child. This guilt stems from the fact that the father is less involved in this drudgery and (secretly and understandably) relieved that it is not he who is bearing the brunt of the problem.

During the early (prepubertal) course of the disease, the patient should be asked what he has been told by his parents, teachers, siblings and peers, and a frank discussion of his concerns initiated. A simple explanation of muscular dystrophy can be given. One must be truthful but optimistic. The patient has to be encouraged to unburden himself of fears and fantasies, and the doctor must be a good listener.

As mentioned, it is desirable to keep the child in a regular school as long as possible. Such a school is usually close to home where the child is permitted to attend with his friends. After-school and vacation activities are thereby enhanced. Such an arrangement requires the cooperation of the principal. A telephone call from the physician can often clarify matters and gain this cooperation.

Preventive psychiatry can be employed, particularly during puberty. At this time fantasies run rampant and should be discussed. Denial and aggression are also apparent in this phase and bear attention. One ought to discuss feelings of dependency on the mother, the need for privacy, and the matter of masturbation. Where a physician feels unprepared or unable to handle these matters, both parents and child should be referred to an appropriate person (psychologist, social worker, psychiatrist) or agency where such help is available.

BIBLIOGRAPHY

Black, F. W. (1973), 'Intellectual Ability as Related to Age and Stage of Disease in Muscular Dystrophy: A Brief Note,' *J. Psychol.*, **84,** 333–334.

Dubowitz, V. (1965), 'Intellectual Impairment in Muscular Dystrophy,' *Arch. Dis. Childh.*, **40,** 296–301.

Marsh, Gayle G. and Munsat, T. L. (1974), 'Evidence for Early Impairment of Verbal Intelligence in Duchenne Muscular Dystrophy,' *Arch. Dis. Childh.*, **49,** No. 2, 118–122.

Rosman, N. P. and Kakulas, B. A. (1966), 'Mental Deficiency Associated with Muscular Dystrophy—A Neuropathological Study,' *Brain*, **89,** 769–787.

Siegel, I. M. and Kornfeld, Marcia S. 'Parental Group Therapy in the Management of a Chronic Fatal Childhood Disease (Duchenne Muscular Dystrophy)—A Combined Medical and Psycho-Social Approach.' Unpublished manuscript.

Steinhauer, P. D., Mushin, D. N. and Rae-Grant, Q. (1974), 'Psychological Aspects of Chronic Illness,' *Pediat. Clin. N. Amer.*, **21,** No. 4, 825–840.

Taft, L. T. (1973), 'The Care and Management of the Child with Muscular Dystrophy,' *Develop. Med. Child. Neurol.*, **15,** 510–518.

Tomonaga, M., Muro, T. and Kito, S. (1967), 'Intelligence Scale and Electroencephalographic Findings on the Progressive Muscular Dystrophy,' *Iryo*, **21,** No. 7, 800–806.

Worden, D. K. and Vignos, P. J., Jr. (1962), 'Intellectual Function in Childhood Progressive Muscular Dystrophy,' *Pediatrics*, **29,** 968–977.

CHAPTER 12

Gradient Measurement of Strength and Functional Ability

Need for Periodic Measurement
  Exercise Management
  Timing of Treatment
  Evaluation Therapy
Modified Muscle Testing
  Strength
  Range of Motion
  Standard Functional Tasks
    Method
    Time
Functional Scale
  Description
  Application

Skeletal muscle comprises 50% of adult weight (25% in the infant) and utilizes 50–70% of the body's metabolism. There are approximately 640 human skeletal muscles ranging in size from the almost miniscule stapedius to the often massive gluteus maximus. There are 250 million skeletal muscle fibres in the body. If all of these fibres contracted maximally at one time, approximately 25 tons of force would be generated. The gastroc-soleus muscle alone can potentially generate 775 pounds of force, and this is because at maximum strength about 42 pounds of force per square inch is generated by normal muscle.

From a rehabilitation standpoint, the net result of muscle weakness, contracture and imbalance determines a patient's ability to perform the activities of daily living. Standard muscle testing which follows changes in strength in individual muscles is not sensitive enough to evaluate the collective functional status of muscle groups, depending as they do on the delicate balance between agonist and antagonist, and the relative activities of those muscles which essentially stabilize position (tonic) and those which mostly activate movement (phasic).

Need

Periodic measurement of strength and function is necessary, not only for the intelligent daily management of activity and exercise in the dystrophic patient, but for timing orthotic, physiatric, and surgical treatment, and evaluating the end result of such therapy. Functional evaluation and modified muscle testing are both necessary if a valid composite picture of overall strength and ability is desired. Serial examination should be conducted no less frequently than at three month intervals.

Testing

Modified muscle testing grades key muscles both as to strength and range of motion against gravity. Thus, with more range of motion, less strength is required for a given task. Any change in range is interpreted as indicative of a change in strength. Because muscle imbalance is as important as specific muscle weakness, this method enables the prescription of exercise programmes designated to relieve such imbalance.

The patient's ability to perform a number of standard tasks is also assessed. Both the time required and the method employed to complete the task are recorded. Subtle alterations in method and even slight changes in time required for any given task objectively reflect changes in strength.

Following is an outline of those muscles and muscle groups routinely measured as to time and method of performance (Charts 9 at end of this chapter).

Functional Scale

Additionally, patients can generally be placed on a functional scale, and the ten-step scale developed by Vignos and his colleagues (modifying the eight-stage classification of Swinyard *et al.*) has been useful as an indirect method of judging functional ability as determined by strength. This scale is as follows:

1. Walks and climbs stairs without assistance.
2. Walks and climbs stairs with aid of railing.

3. Walks and climbs stairs slowly with aid of railing.
4. Walks but cannot climb stairs.
5. Walks unassisted but cannot climb stairs or get out of chair.
6. Walks only with assistance or with braces.
7. In wheelchair. Sits erect, can roll chair and perform bed and wheelchair activities of daily living.
8. In wheelchair. Sits erect. Unable to perform bed and chair activities without assistance.
9. In wheelchair. Sits erect only with support. Able to do only minimal activities of daily living.
10. In bed. Cannot perform activities of daily living without assistance.

Timing is vital in planning treatment in muscular dystrophy. The indications and conditions for each therapeutic procedure must be met. Although function is of prime concern, comfort and cosmesis are important ancillary considerations. Some applications of the foregoing methods of assessment to the management of patients with muscle disease follow.

In stages 1, 2, and 3 of the Vignos classification, because the patient is ambulating independently (though with a disturbed gait pattern), passive stretch of early lower extremity contractures is necessary, but a programme of specialized exercises is unnecessary as the functional activities of ambulation and daily living are sufficient exercise for these patients. Note that normal five or six-year-olds often use railing assistance while ascending stairs. This makes it sometimes difficult to accurately classify small children into class 1 or 2. Somewhere between stages 5 and 6, lower extremity surgery is indicated because of increase in contracture and difficulty with antigravity activities. Surgery and bracing are necessary as the patient is about to lose his ability to maintain the upright posture at this time. However, such bracing is an encumbrance during the early stages of muscular dystrophy and is prescribed only toward the end of independent ambulation (between stages 5 and 6). This need becomes imminent when the patient begins to require upper extremity support (holding on to furniture, walls, doors, etc.) during ambulation.

Unfortunately, well-meaning parents or teachers sometimes encourage ambulant patients in stages 5 or 6 to avoid activity and to use wheelchairs. Patients so treated lose strength rapidly and become permanently wheelchair-bound within a relatively short period of time.

There is also an unfortunate tendency in some cases to avoid the wheelchair entirely in stage 7, condemning the patient to stage 10 (bed rest) immediately. If properly managed, patients can be taught wheelchair transfer techniques and allowed relative independence for a significantly longer period of time.

When stage 7 is reached, routine conditioning exercises are prescribed to retard diffuse atrophy and keep the patient independent in wheelchair activities as long as possible. It is also essential that patients in stages 7 through 10 be given care appropriate to their physiological needs. This may include use of the tilt table or appropriate bracing and continued contracture stretching. Cardiac and pulmonary problems (also obesity) become more severe during and after stage 7. The closer the patient is to bed confinement, the more assistive devices he requires. Scoliosis is usually only a problem after stage 7.

When plotting changes in functional ability against age, one clearly notes the rapidly declining course in Duchenne dystrophy, as contrasted with the adult myopathies.

In summary, the testing techniques described above are readily learned by any competent therapist, and when performed at three month intervals, provide a reproducible and objective record of functional status and strength, demonstrating progress, or lack of progress of the disease, documenting or anticipating serious change in functional ability, and indicating the need for specific therapies.

BIBLIOGRAPHY

Archibald, K. C. and Vignos, P. J., Jr. (1959), 'A Study of Contractures in Muscular Dystrophy,' *Arch. Phys. Med. Rehab.*, **40,** 150–157.

Daniels, Lucille, Williams, Marian and Worthingham, Catherine (1974), *Muscle Testing—Techniques of Manual Examination.* W. B. Saunders.

Gordon, E. E. and Texidor, T. A. (1964), 'Problems in Muscle Biopsy; An Experimental Study,' *Arch. Phys. Med. Rehab.*, **45,** 396–402.

Miller, Jo. (1964), 'Assessment in the Treatment of Muscle Disease (A Preliminary Report),' *Tex. Rep. Biol. Med.*, **22,** suppl. No. 1, 871–879.

Chart 9A. Modified Muscle Testing and Goniometry

Left									Right							
								Date								
								Therapist								
								Neck flexors								
								Abdominals								
								Scapular winging								
								Shoulder abduction								
								Shoulder extension								
								Elbow flexion								
								Elbow extension								
								Wrist extension								
								Hip extension								
								Hip abduction								
								Hip flexion								
								Knee extension								
								Knee flexion								
								Foot dorsiflexion								
								Foot plantar flexion								
								Foot eversion								
								Foot inversion								
								*Pseudohypertrophy measurement								

*Circumference at widest part of calf.

Left *Right*

								Contractures								
								Hip								
								TFL								
								Knee								
								Ankle								
								Elbow								
								Lag								
								Hip								
								Knee								
								Total								

Explanation of Testing Procedures Modified Muscle Testing

Anterior Neck Musculature

Patient is supine on table. Flexes neck. Resist on forehead and grade *normal* to *fair*. If patient does not have ability to flex antigravity, test sidelying and grade poor to zero.

Abdominal Musculature

Patient is supine on table with knees flexed and feet held by therapist. He attempts to sit up with hands behind head for normal grade (four to five full sit-ups), arms folded across chest for good, arms extended at sides for fair. If patient is unable to do full sit-up in fair position, measure in inches the distance he is able to lift the seventh cervical vertebra from surface and palpate abdominal muscles.

Note: If anterior neck musculature is poor, support head to test for abdominal strength.

Scapular Winging

The patient is sitting and an attempt is made to lift patient at both axillas. If the patient 'slips through' and the scapulae becomes more prominent, it indicates a weakness of the serratus anterior and other shoulder girdle musculature. This should be marked 'yes' or 'no' on the form.

Shoulder Abduction

Patient sits straight with arms at sides, then, with palms down, raises arms to sides and over head bilaterally to avoid substitution. Do not allow patient to come into flexion. If patient has full range of motion, resist at elbows to 90° abduction and grade *normal* to *fair*. If patient has less than full antigravity range of motion, measure the degree of motion with the goniometer axis at the shoulder joint, using a line parallel to the midline of the body for one arm, the midline of the humerus for the other.

If patient has no antigravity motion, test in the supine position and grade from poor to zero.

Shoulder extension

Patient is prone on table, arm over edge and shoulder flexed to 90°. Extends shoulder with palm up while scapula is stablized. If patient has full range of antigravity motion, measure the angle, calling 90° of shoulder flexion (starting position) 0° extension and measuring up toward full extension (approximately 125°) down the midline of the humerus toward lateral epicondyle with axis at the shoulder joint. Give assistance at elbow at neutral position (90° extension from starting position) and grade *normal* to *fair*. If patient has less than full range of antigravity motion, measure angle of extension as described above. Resist as able. If patient has no antigravity extension, measure sidelying and grade poor to zero.

Elbow Flexion

Patient sits with arms at sides, elbows fully extended, then flexes one elbow; may use all elbow flexors. If patient has full range of motion, give resistance at wrist and grade *normal* to *fair*. If patient lacks full range against gravity, elbow may be set in initial flexion to achieve full range; this is then noted. If patient has no antigravity flexion, position supine and attempt elbow flexion, grading poor to zero.

Elbow Extension

Patient is prone on table, arm over edge and shoulder flexed to 90°. Extends shoulder with palm up while scapula is stablized. If patient has full range of antigravity motion, give resistance at wrist and grade *normal* to *fair*. If patient has less than full range, measure from 90° flexion to degree of extensor lag using lateral epicondyle as axis and aligning one arm with greater tubercle of humerus, the other with radial head and record 90 to degree of lag as active motion (example 90–20°). If patient has no antigravity extension, position supine and grade poor to zero.

Wrist Extension

Patient sits with elbow flexed to 90°, extends wrist with fingers relaxed. If patient has full range of motion, antigravity, give resistance to extension and grade *normal* to *fair*. If patient has less than full antigravity motion, grade fair minus. If patient lacks antigravity motion, attempt extension with hand supported on ulnar border and grade poor to zero.

Hip Extension

Patient is prone over edge of table with trunk supported, hips flexed to 90°, knees extended and feet on floor. Keeping knee straight, patient extends hip through range. If patient has full range of antigravity motion, resist at knee and grade *normal* to *fair*. If patient has less than full range, measure the degree of hip extension from 90° flexion through range, using greater trochanter as axis and the midline of the trunk and lateral condyle of femur as sights for the goniometer arms. Record (example, 90–30°, 60° active motion). Resist as able. If patient has no antigravity hip extension, position sidelying and grade poor to zero.

Note: If patient has full range of motion, may also test prone on the table and extend hip with knee extended and grade *normal* to *fair*.

Hip Abduction

Patient is in the sidelying position with the leg slightly extended beyond the midline. The patient abducts the leg through range of motion for fair grade; resist at the knee for good to normal. Poor grade is tested in supine position.

Hip Flexion

The patient is sitting with both knees flexed to 90°. Patient flexes one hip through range of motion for fair grade; resist at the knee for good to normal. Poor grade muscle is tested in sidelying position with upper leg supported, patient flexes hip through range of motion.

Knee Extension

Patient sits with hip and knee flexed to 90°, hands in lap. Extends knee through range of motion while maintaining erect posture. If patient has full range, give resistance at ankle and grade *normal* to *fair*. If patient lacks full range, measure from 90° flexion to limit of extension using lateral condyle of femur as axis with one arm of goniometer aligned with greater trochanter, the other with lateral malleolus. Record extensor lag and degree of motion (example 90–30°, 60° active motion). Resist as able and grade. If patient has no antigravity extension, test in sidelying and grade poor to zero.

Knee Flexion

The patient is supine and flexes knee through range of motion for fair grade. Resist for good to normal. Poor grade is tested with patient sidelying and upper leg supported, patient flexes knee.

Foot Dorsiflexion

Patient is supine on table. From position of planter flexion, he dorsiflexes and resistance is given on dorsal aspect of foot; grade *normal* to *fair*. If patient lacks full range, grade fair minus. If patient has no antigravity dorsiflexion, position sidelying and grade poor to zero.

Foot Plantar Flexion

Tested with patient standing and being able to stand on toes of the foot for good to normal grade. Fair grade is tested with patient prone and foot extended over edge of table at 90°, patient plantar flexes foot.

Foot Eversion

Tested with patient supine. Patient everts foot from plantar flexed position. Resist at lateral border of foot for good to normal grade. Tested sidelying for fair grade, and patient everts foot through range of motion.

Foot Inversion

Tested in supine position. Patient inverts foot through range of motion for fair grade; resist at medial border of forefoot for good to normal grades.

Measurement of Contractures

Hip flexion Contracture

Measure in Thomas position, one knee flexed to chest, allowing no lordosis, extend other leg avoiding any abduction. Measure along midline of trunk and toward lateral femoral condyle with axis of goniometer at greater trochanter.

Tensor Fascia Lata Tightness

Measure prone with leg abducted to eliminate as much hip flexion contracture as possible and cause maximum relaxation of tensor. Flex knee to 90°, exert pressure on sacrum and adduct leg until hip flexes further. Measure angle of abduction with one arm of goniometer on posterior iliac spines, other arm extending down midline of posterior aspect of leg.

Knee Flexion Contracture

Measure with patient supine, legs extended to greatest degree possible, using lateral femoral condyle as axis and sighting to greater trochanter and lateral malleolus.

Plantar Flexion Contracture

Measure in test position for foot dorsiflexion. Exert pressure on plantar surface of foot to insure maximum passive dorsiflexion. Measure laterally along fibula and plantar surface of foot. Record dorsiflexion of plantar flexion contracture.

Elbow Flexion Contracture

Measure in test position for elbow extension, assist to full passive extension when necessary. Place arms of goniometer along midline of humerus and radius as described under testing procedures for elbow extension.

Chart 9B. Functional Assessment Chart

Name:											
Activity	*Date*										
	Therapist										
		Time to Accomplish Task									
1. Run 25 feet											
2. Walk 25 feet	a. independent										
	b. short leg braces										
	c. long leg braces										
	d. crutches, walker or cane										
3. Climb 8 stairs	a. independent—foot over foot										
	b. independent—one step at a time										
	c. hands on knees										
	d. railing—one hand										
	e. railing and hand on knee										
	f. railing—two hands										
4. Walk down 8 stairs	a. independent										
	b. railing—one hand										
	c. railing—two hands										

5. Rise from chair	a. independent										
	b. Gower's sign										
	c. turn to side, then push up										
	d. pull up with aid of table										
6. Roll over from supine to prone											
7. Roll over from prone to supine											
8. Get to all-fours position from prone											
9. Sit up from	a. independent										
Supine	b. pull up										
	c. pull up and push on elbows										
	d. turn to side, then push up										
	e. to hand and knees, then sit up										
10. Rise from floor	a. independent										
from prone	b. Gower's sign										
position	c. chair to standing										
	d. chair to sitting, then to standing										
11. Sitting balance	a. stable										
	b. unstable										
12. Vital capacity—	sitting										
13. Height											
14. Weight											
15. Hand grip	a. right										
	b. left										

Explanation of Testing Procedures
Functional Assessment Chart

ACTIVITY—timed (1 through 10) and observed (11)

1. **Run 25 feet**
   Both feet off the ground at one time.

2. **Walk 25 feet**
   a. independent—no assistance from mechanical aids.
   b. short leg braces—test items 3, 4, and 5 with braces also.
   c. long leg braces—test items 3, 4, and 5 with braces also.
   d. crutches, walker or cane.

Stair measurements: Depth—$11\frac{1}{2}''$; height—7″; railing height—36″.

3. **Climb 8 stairs**
   a. independent—foot over foot—no assistance such as pushing on knee, using rail.
   b. independent—one step at a time.
   c. hands on knees—assistance from rail.
   d. railing—one hand.
   e. railing and hand on knee—patient pulls on rail with one hand, pushes on knee with the other.
   f. railing—two hands, some patients may use two rails.

4. **Walk down 8 stairs**
   a. independent—no assistance from rail. May go foot over foot, or one step at a time.
   b. railing—one hand, often used for safety but not for support.
   c. railing—two hands, or rail and therapist's hand for safety.

5. **Rise from chair**
   Care must be taken to seat the patient in a chair which places his feet flat on the floor and his knees in 90° flexion. This is particularly important with children as a higher chair would give them a mechanical advantage.

   a. independent—rising without pushing on chair or knees, arms folded across chest or extended.
   b. Gower's sign—includes pressure on knees or pressure on seat of chair or both.
   c. turn to side, then push up—patient turns sideways in chair to sit on one hip, with feet on floor pushes with arms to 90° hip flexion and pushes off to upright position or climbs up chair to upright position.
   d. pull up with aid of table—patient takes support from table with hips flexed while extending knees. Once knees are locked, patient extends hips by pushing up on table.

6. **Roll over from supine to prone**
   Contractures may inhibit this activity.

7. **Roll over from prone to supine**
   Contractures may inhibit this activity.

8. **Get to all-fours position from prone**
   Push up to hands and knees.

9. **Sit up from supine**
   a. independent—no aids other than having ankles held down by therapist which is within the range of normal; must achieve sitting balance.
   b. pull up—patient holds on to leg or clothing to pull himself up.
   c. pull and push on elbow—begins to pull up, then pushes on at least one elbow.
   d. turn to side, then push up—patient will roll to side, then push up with both arms to achieve sitting balance.
   e. to hands and knees, then sit up—roll to prone, to hands and knees, then to side sit or other sitting balance.

10. **Rise from floor from prone position**
    a. independent—no assistance required.
    b. Gower's sign—can bring himself to his feet but must push on knees to assume erect posture.
    c. chair to standing—patient pulls himself to feet with aid of chair, then pushes on chair to achieve upright position.
    d. chair to sitting, then to standing—patient pulls himself to sitting position in chair, then pushes himself to upright position, using chair.

Patient should be placed on edge of table with thighs fully supported and knees flexed to 90°.

11. **Sitting balance**
    a. stable.
    b. unstable—patient sits erect but cannot recover balance if it is lost. Or, patient is unable to maintain his balance without support of his arms.

12. **Vital capacity**
    Measured sitting, taking highest of two readings. Take height and weight into consideration.

13. **Height.**

14. **Weight.**

15. **Hand grip**
    Measured with Newman myometer taking highest of two readings for left and right hands. Keep arms at side during measurement.

CHAPTER 13

Pathomechanics

Duchenne dystrophics provide an excellent opportunity for studying postural pathomechanics secondary to muscular weakness, tendon contracture, and mechanical malposture. The problems of deformity in the milder and/or later occurring forms of muscular dystrophy are also similar to those in the Duchenne patient.

Biomechanical Sequence

Following is an outline of the biomechanical sequence leading to the typical dystrophic posture of lumbar lordosis, hip abduction and flexion, knee flexion, ankle equinus, and calcaneocavovarus of the feet. It should be understood that these events overlap in occurrence and many take place concurrently.

1. Weakness of hip extensors and shoulder stabilizers.
2. Hip flexor contracture forcing trunk forward.
3. Compensatory lumbar lordosis (Fig. 29).
4. Due to forward shift of centre of mass, patient rises on his toes, thus shortening the ankle to toes lever arm and shifting centre of gravity forward.
5. Hip abduction increases equilibrium by widening the body's base of support (Fig. 30). Proprioceptive input may be affected by failure of muscle spindle function resulting from altered physical state of skeletal muscle giving support to muscle spindle. This also

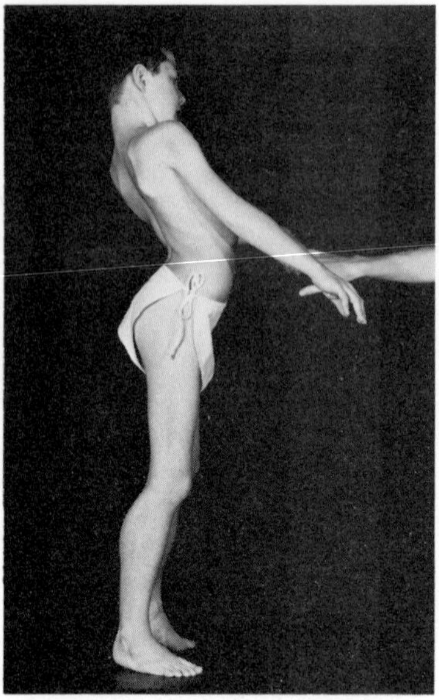

Fig. 29. Compensatory lumbar lordosis.

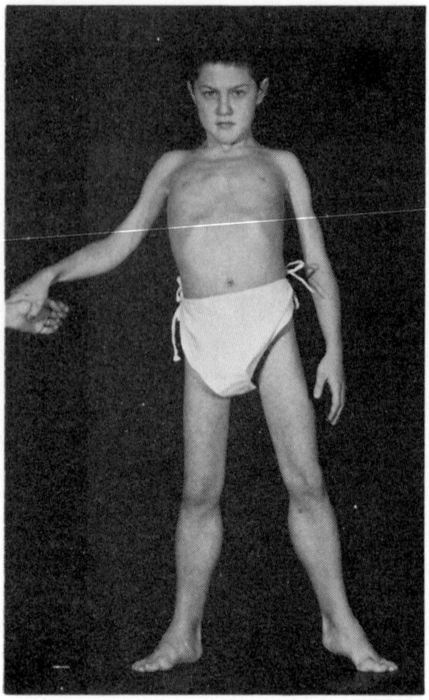

Fig. 30. Increased hip abduction for equilibrium.

contributes to the disappearance of the deep tendon reflexes.

6. Contracture of the tensor fascia lata.

7. External tibial torsion; thus ankle and knee axes are no longer in the same plane.

8. Ankle varus (an effort to bring ankle into better postural alignment) (Fig. 31).

9. Knee flexion for balance.

10. Quadriceps weakens; equinus required to lock knees for stability.

11. With foot fixed and knee flexed, gastrocnemius-soleus now acts to extend knee.

12. True exercise hypertrophy of calf as it overworks to maintain the knee in extension. This is a compensatory hypertrophy in postural muscles (calves, quadriceps, gluteals, lower paravertebral musculature, and even serratus anterior). This hypertrophy develops in response to a postural demand with a resultant dynamic equinus and is the first step on the road to atrophy (Fig. 32).

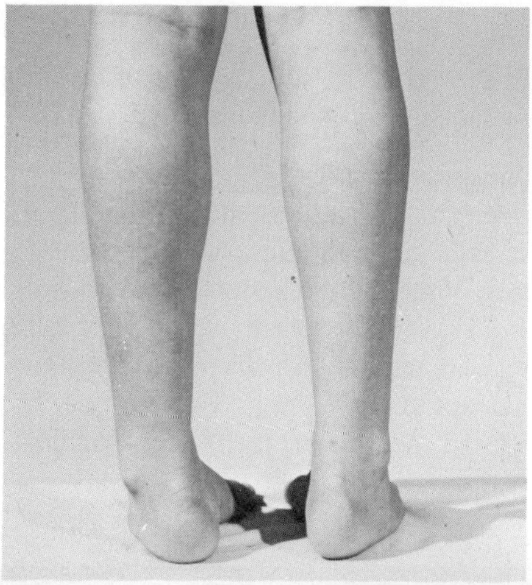

Fig. 31. Increase in ankle varus.

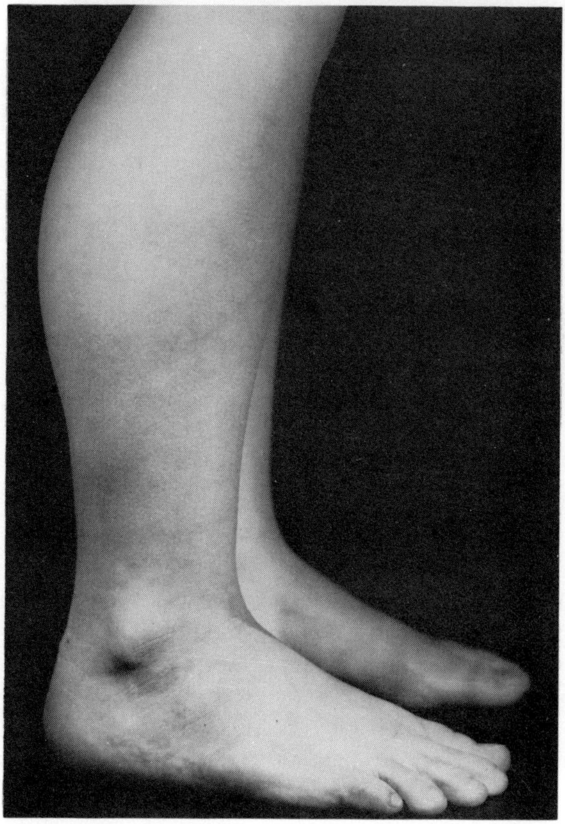

Fig. 32. Exercise hypertrophy of calves.

13. Widening of base of support with concomitant increase of those forces causing equinocavovarus (Fig. 33):

a. Unopposed heel cord contracture acting upon eccentric medial insertion of Achilles tendon.
b. Tarsal slide in an anterior medial direction.
c. Increase of toe flexion action for grasp stability.
d. Secondary intrinsic foot muscle contracture.
e. Unopposed action of tibialis posticus against weak peroneals and tibialis anticus.
f. Unopposed action of toe flexors against weakened toe extensors.

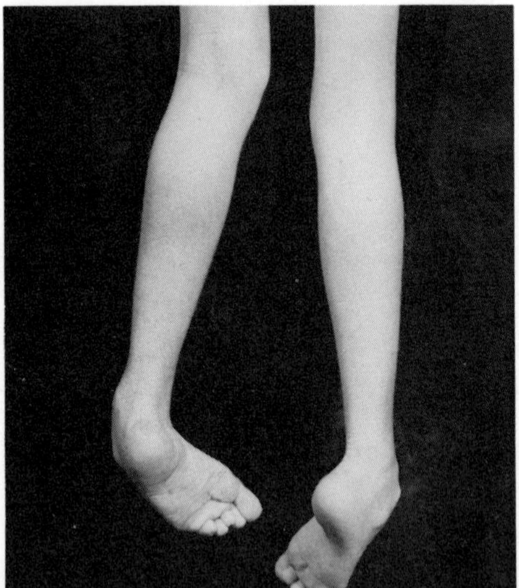

Fig. 33.

14. Triceps surae overwork stress with 'pseudohypertrophy'. Those muscles or muscle groups required to maintain posture, provide mechanical support, or subject to any constant deforming regional stretch, undergo profound atrophy. The postural muscles may develop hypertrophy prior to this, but ultimately this physiological increase in muscle size is followed by the production of a free fat staining substance, reactive fibrosis, and eventual

lipomatosis of the muscle mass. This is known as pseudohypertrophy. It is dependent upon an intact lower motor neuron, and in cases of poliomyelitis superimposed on muscular dystrophy, it disappears.

The net result of these events is a stance and gait typified by lumbar lordosis, hip flexion and abduction, knee flexion, ankle equinus, and calcaneocavovarus of the feet (Fig. 34).

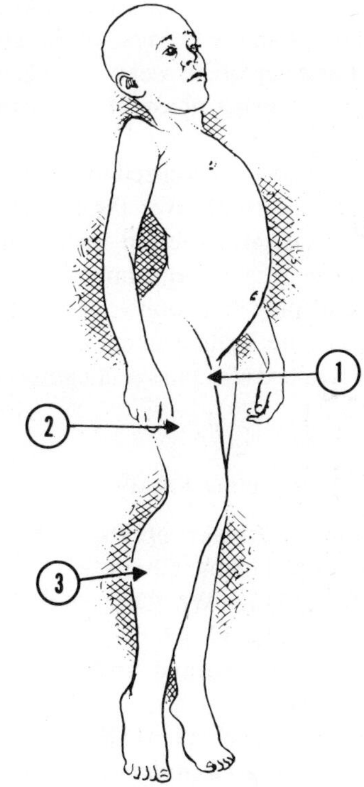

Fig. 34. Stance and gait typified by lumbar lordosis due to (1) hip flexion, (2) hip abduction, knee flexion with ankle equinus secondary to contracture of (3) Achilles tendon and calcaneocavovarus of the feet.

Line of Gravity

Such patients fall because as hip extensor weakness progresses, increased lumbar lordosis becomes necessary to keep the line of gravity behind the hips. However, this line of gravity must, at the same time, be maintained in front of the knee. Hip flexion contracture (including tensor fasciae lata) blocks this manoeuvre by preventing hip extension and causing knee flexion. Even hyperextending the neck, using the head to sustain the weight line, is insufficient to maintain upright posture, as the patient comes up on his toes to help keep the hips and knees extended. Additionally, progressive quadriceps weakness makes knee stability difficult.

Another mechanism which may cause falling is the development of mediolateral subtalar instability because of the above noted muscular imbalance (strong posterior tibial, weak peroneals, etc.), allowing the foot to invert during the swing phase of gait with initiation of stance in this insecure position.

As the disease progresses, generalized weakness makes it increasingly difficult to balance the trunk over the unstable lower extremities. Proprioceptive abilities are also affected. Such patients require strength enough to execute those postural adjustments necessary to compensate for their selective weakening and contracture. In this regard small non-muscular changes assume significance. A slight gain in weight or a period of several days of bed rest can significantly decrease strength and prohibit ambulation.

BIBLIOGRAPHY

Bonsett, C. A. (1969), *Studies of Pseudohypertrophic Muscular Dystrophy*. Springfield, Illinois: Charles C. Thomas.

Merton, P. A. (1972), 'How We Control the Contraction of Our Muscles,' *Sci. Amer.*, **226,** 30–37.

Rosenthal, A. M. (1969), 'Normal and Abnormal Gait Patterns,' *Illinois med. J.*, **136,** 50–54.

Siegel, I. M. (1972), 'Pathomechanics of Stance in Duchenne Muscular Dystrophy,' *Arch. Phys. Med. Rehab.*, **53,** 403–406.

CHAPTER 14

General Principles of Orthopaedic Treatment

There should be no apathy toward the rehabilitation of patients with muscular dystrophy because physicians and therapists bear a medical and moral responsibility to do everything possible for their welfare. While research is seeking the cause and cure of these diseases, a rehabilitation programme should strive to make them as self-sufficient as possible, both physically and vocationally, and offer psycho-social support appropriate to the changing phases of their illness.

Some types of muscle disease progress very slowly indeed, and by providing self-help devices and preventing deformities, it is possible to keep these patients vocationally occupied and well adjusted for many years beyond the time they might be so without such assistance.

Finally, until a specific cure is discovered, all attempts to treat muscular dystrophy will be palliative. Nonetheless, it is desirable to preserve maximal physical function pending such discovery because when it is possible to arrest the disease process, those patients ambulatory will be in better stead than those confined to a wheelchair, who in turn will be better off than those in bed.

Thus, an aggressive programme of early diagnosis, general care, genetic counselling, supportive physiatry, psychologic counselling, assistive devices, prophylaxis and treatment of respiratory and cardiac problems, surgery, and bracing are important in maintaining residual function. Developing and perfecting techniques to do this, represents a continuing challenge to medicine.

General Principles

Physical therapy is directed toward:

1. Improving muscular strength.
2. Preventing and correcting contractures.
3. Increasing efficiency of functional activities of daily living.

One must decide whether the disease process is progressive, recurrent or static. If significant regeneration of muscle fibres can yet occur (inflammatory myopathy), treatment will produce greater benefit.

Orthopaedic treatment aimed at the prevention and correction of contracture and deformity and the provision of support through assistive orthoses leads to the maintenance of maximal function of the whole patient.

Deformities

Three processes contribute concurrently to the deformities of muscular dystrophy:

1. Specific muscle weakness.
2. Muscle imbalance (agonist versus antagonist).
3. Specific muscle contracture (secondary to gravity and compensatory postural habitus).

Therefore, it is necessary to strengthen weak musculature and stretch contracted muscles so that muscular imbalance will not lead to diffuse atrophy. Orthoses, such as pelvic bands, are usually unnecessary, as are back supports, such as the Knight spinal attachment. Night splints are generally used. Such splintage should be in addition to and not instead of manual contracture stretching. These splints are best employed prophylactically. They are of little value after deformities have occurred. Short leg night splints for ankle equinus may initiate or increase knee flexion contracture due to the tendency of patients to flex their knees in order to relieve discomfort from gastrocnemius tightness. Long leg splints are advised.

It is important to maintain alignment support in the body, and stretching (particularly of heel cord contractures) is vital as severe equinus can make the difference between walking or not. In addition to ankle equinus, hip flexion contracture, tensor fasciae contracture (as well as contracture of gluteus medius and minimus) and knee flexion contracture should be avoided where possible and stretched when present.

In the adult (milder) myopathies (such as dystrophia myotonica and facioscapulohumeral dystrophy) heel cord contracture can be managed with a spring-wire-drop-foot-brace, or a floor reaction orthoses (Fig. 35). Massage, electrical stimulation, etc., are ineffective in the treatment of advancing muscular weakness, imbalance and contracture.

Patients with Duchenne dystrophy suffer severe atrophy of disuse when put to bed. They should not be bed or chair-confined for more than a day at most. The usual diseases of childhood, including the exanthems, can often be managed without complication while allowing the patient ambulatory privileges.

Standing and walking are the best functional physical therapy for the patient with muscular dystrophy. However, alternate standing should be encouraged to avoid heel cord contracture. Most people stand in a position of haunch, with one foot habitually advanced (Fig. 36). This extremity develops heel cord and hip flexion contracture early because the child prefers the better aligned limb. This side is stretched while the opposite undergoes progressive contracture. Active (functional) exercises can retard disuse atrophy during the early phases of the disease and are effective as ongoing treatment in the adult dystrophies where they can result in muscle strengthening. When these fail, active assisted and passive stretch exercising can be employed (Chart 10). Surgery (contracture release) and bracing are delayed until conservative

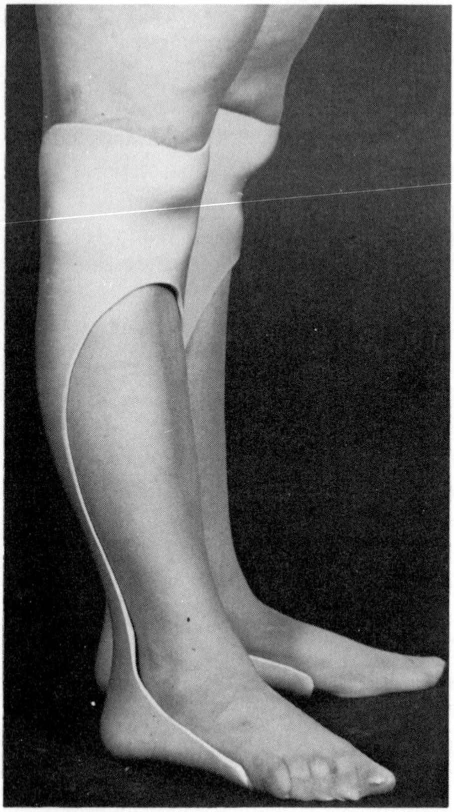

Fig. 35. Floor reaction orthosis designed to correct foot drop.

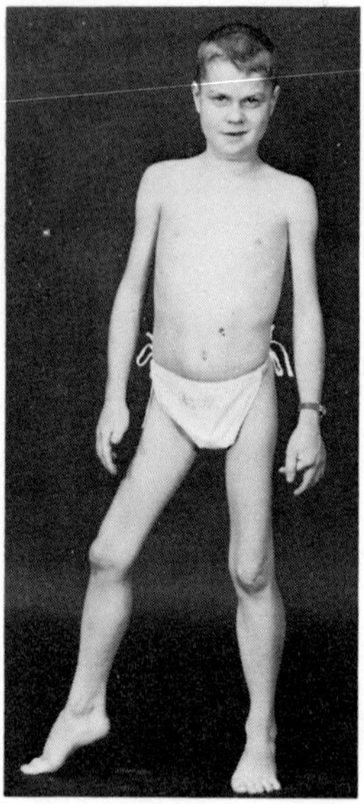

Fig. 36. Haunch-posture with one foot advanced. This extremity develops early heel cord contracture, as illustrated.

measures are no longer effective.

It is common to find children with long-standing muscle disease whose severe secondary deformities are a much greater handicap than the primary muscle weakness. Although weakening is symmetrical in many of the muscular dystrophies, joint contractures are not so. Unequal contracture is due to habitually maintained postures, both awake and asleep, and also to increased activity in the dominant extremities, retarding the development of and reducing contractures already formed. It is mostly those muscles which span two joints that contract the earliest and the most. One cannot prevent primary weakness, but atrophy of disuse and contracture should be avoidable.

Chart 10. Exercises for Stretching Key Musculature

Muscles	*Active*	*Passive*
(1) Hip Flexors	Lying supine at edge of bed or table, hold opposite knee and hip flexed, drop leg over edge and allow weight of extremity to extend hip.	Patient prone—knees extended—while stabilizing hip from behind elevate knee from the table.
(2) Tensor Fascia (iliotibial band)	Stand with one side toward wall and feet about 8–12 inches from the wall. Keep knees straight and lean the near hip toward the wall.	Patient prone, thigh extended and abducted. Stabilizing hip posteriorly adduct hip to maximum stretch position.
(3) Hamstrings	Toe-touching in standing or seated position with the knees straight.	Patient supine, hip flexed, knee extended, elevate leg to maximum stretch position.
(4) Heel Cords	Stand arms length from a wall. Supporting body with hands on wall and keeping knees extended and *heels on the floor* attempt to lean chest to wall, thus dorsiflexing ankles.	Patient supine, knees extended. Cup heel in palm, maintaining foot in neutral position and supporting sole to avoid bending foot at tarsal joints. Dorsiflex ankle to position of maximal stretch.

Maintenance of ambulation also leads to less soft tissue atrophy, less severe osteoporosis and better circulation. Movement at night is prevented by severe flexion contracture, and preserving joint mobility increases the patient's ability to turn independently during sleep. The psychological benefits of the upright posture and the ability to ambulate require no comment. It has been reported that children standing less than two hours daily have an increase in heel cord contracture due to flexor-extensor muscle imbalance, and a concurrent decrease in strength due to diffuse muscle atrophy. The use of the standing table, both at school and at home, gives such children standing time, so that the tendency to develop lower extremity contracture can be decreased. As Lewin so aptly stated, 'Position is everything in the life of a limb'.

Although adequate functional exercise and active stretching by the patient himself are important in maintaining residual strength and mobility in patients with muscular dystrophy, fatique must be avoided. Heavy exercise increases serum CPK, and this may initiate accelerated degradation of residual muscle.

Obesity can be a serious problem in the management of muscular dystrophy. It occurs because the patient's food intake is far in excess of his reduced energy demand. This is a particular problem when the child becomes wheelchair-bound, because of a combination of psychic overeating (often a technique to handle anxiety), parental pampering, and minimal energy demands while confined to a chair.

Assistive Devices

A variety of mechanical, assistive devices significantly aid in the care of the dystrophic child. Wheelchairs will be discussed separately. Patients with weak quadriceps muscles function better when they use chairs (and toilet seats) which are raised. This enables the child to rise and sit independently, or, at least, with a minimum of help. Older children and adults may benefit by a chair which either electrically or mechanically lifts them to the standing position (e.g. orthokinetic lift chair). A bathtub stool used with a shower spray allows the patient to bathe in the tub with decreased physical strain on his back. Grab bars are helpful in the bathroom. A crib-size hospital bed with side rails enables a child to turn more easily. The additional height even permits some patients to get out of bed independently.

Clothing adaptations for the child with progressive muscular dystrophy, utilizing special zippers on trousers, easily manipulated

Velcro fastenings, etc., have facilitated independence and self care. Socks, one size too large with elastic tops, and an oversized, buttoned shirt are easier to don than clothing which fits perfectly. Shoes should have low heels (or be negatively heeled) to avoid encouraging equinus contracture of the heel cords.

Foot boards to diminish heel cord contracture, and over-bed cradles to keep covers off the legs are recommended. Such a cradle enables the patient to move more freely in bed without fighting the weight of blankets. This is particularly helpful in winter. Sleeping in the prone position is encouraged to keep hip flexors stretched. Electronic, hydraulic, or mechanical lifts are useful for transferring to and from a bath or bed. For those who cannot turn themselves at night, an alternating pressure mattress, 'waffled' foam rubber mattress, or sheep-skin

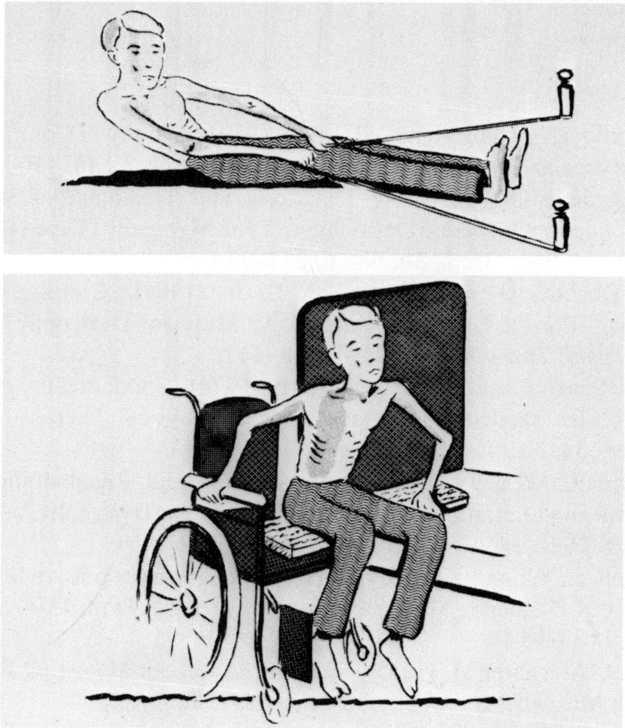

Fig. 37. *Above:* Clothesline used as aid in rising to sitting position.
Below: Sliding transfer board used in moving from chair to bed.

pads have been helpful in either facilitating movement or avoiding pressure irritation.

Residual muscles are used more effectively within a limited range of motion, and, therefore, long-handled utensils (toilet articles, eating utensils) are more easily manipulated than those of standard size. A length of smooth cord (clothesline), tied to the end of the bed, provides a simple rig to aid a child in rising to the sitting position. A transfer board, upon which the patient can slide, facilitates moving from bed to chair, or vice-versa (Fig. 37). The use of nylon or satin sheets decrease body-bedclothes friction, making changing bed position easier. A variety of suggestions, techniques, and descriptions of apparatus to aid in the daily care of the dystrophic child have been published in several pamphlets by the Muscular Dystrophy Association, Inc.

BIBLIOGRAPHY

Archibald, K. C. and Vignos, P. J., Jr. (1959), 'A Study of Contractures in Muscular Dystrophy,' *Arch. Phys. Med. Rehab.*, **40,** 150–157.

Demos, Jean (1971), 'Early Diagnosis and Treatment of Rapidly Developing Duchenne DeBoulogne Type Myopathy (Type DDB 1),' *Amer. J. Phys. Med.*, **50,** No. 6, 271–284.

Hall, Dorothy S. and Vignos, P. J., Jr. (1964), 'Clothing Adaptions—For the Child with Progressive Muscular Dystrophy,' *Amer. J. Occup. Ther.*, **XVIII,** No. 3, 108–112.

Harris, Susan E. and Cherry, Dianne B. (1974), 'Childhood Progressive Muscular Dystrophy and the Role of Physical Therapy,' *Phys. Ther.*, **54,** No. 1, 4–12.

Hoberman, M. (1955), 'Physical Medicine and Rehabilitation: Its Value and Limitations in Progressive Muscular Dystrophy,' *Amer. J. Phys. Med.*, **34,** 109–115.

Johnson, E. W. and Kennedy, J. H. (1971), 'Comprehensive Management of Duchenne Muscular Dystrophy,' *Arch. Phys. Med. Rehab.*, **52,** 110–114.

Kenrick, Margaret M. (1965), 'Certain Aspects of Managing Patients with Muscular Dystrophy,' *Sth. med. J.*, **58,** No. 2, 996–1000.

Paul, W. D. (1954), 'Medical Management of Contractures in Muscular Dystrophy,' *Symposium on Contracture of Muscle.* Third Medical Conference, Muscular Dystrophy Associations of America, Incorporated, New York.

Swinyard, C. A., Deaver, G. G. and Greenspan, L. (1958), *Progressive Muscular Dystrophy Diagnosis and Problems of Rehabilitation.* Scientific Department, Muscular Dystrophy Associations of America, Incorporated.

Vignos, P. J., Jr. (1968), 'Rehabilitation in Progressive Muscular Dystrophy,' in *Rehabilitation and Medicine*, pp. 584–642 (S. Licht, Ed.) New London: CT. E. Licht.

Vignos, P. J., Jr. and Watkins, Mary P. (1966), 'The Effect of Exercise in Muscular Dystrophy,' *J. Amer. Med. Ass.*, **197,** 843–848.

Wratney, Martha J. (1958), 'Physical Therapy for Muscular Dystrophy Children,' *Phys. Ther. Rev.*, **38,** No. 1. 26–32.

CHAPTER 15

Surgical Treatment: Hip and Ankle Deformity

Timing

To paraphrase Steindler, 'Surgery is but one moment in the total treatment of the child with muscular dystrophy'. However, in few conditions is the timing of the moment as important a consideration as in the elective surgery of this disease.

As concerns ambulation, lower extremity contractures increase until the unstable base of support secondary to equinovarus and the pelvic imbalance produced by hip flexion contracture prohibit walking. Surgery cannot be delayed beyond this point, because with rare exception, once a patient becomes wheelchair-bound, he will not walk again.

For this reason it is essential to recognize the signs of early difficulty in walking and to correct deformities impeding balance so that ambulation can be prolonged. At the same time, surgical procedures designed to do this must not require prolonged bedrest, or entail excessive pain, as such measures would defeat themselves by restraining the patient in bed.

Deforming Forces

The muscles developing ambulation limiting contractures in the lower extremities are:

1. Hip flexors.
2. Tensor fasciae latae.
3. Triceps surae.

As quadriceps weakness progresses and contracture increases in these muscle groups, the base of support decreases and, in trying to balance, the child walks with a wide gait, characterized by equinus, heel varus, knee flexion and hip flexion and abduction (Fig. 38).

Increased lumbar lordosis is noted early as an attempt to compensate for pelvic imbalance secondary to weakened hip extension accom-

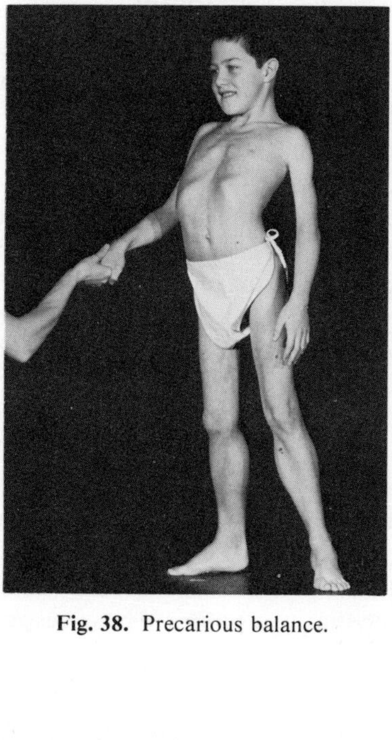

Fig. 38. Precarious balance.

panied by hip flexion contracture. Abdominal and low back extensor weakness contribute to the grotesque and effortful gait, and loss of strength in the shoulder depressors makes torso balance awkward. Parascapular weakening draws the shoulders forward, increasing the need for lumbar lordosis to achieve torso balance.

Aims

The aims of leg surgery are (1) to release lower extremity contractures sufficiently to bring the body into adequate standing and walking equilibrium and (2) to strengthen the lower limbs so that light-weight braces can be applied for support.

Generally speaking, bracing and the surgery necessary to place the lower limbs into braces is advised when, due to a combination of both weakness and contracture, balance becomes precarious and the patient begins to find walking increasingly difficult. This is usually heralded by more frequent loss of balance and falling. As a rule of thumb, loss of functional ability to rise from the floor, climb stairs and walk are lost at approximate intervals of one year in the order stated.

Assessment

Muscle strength assessment by functional testing and serial measurement of joint contracture aid in determining when such surgery is necessary. With few exceptions, with equinovarus deformity present and a combined knee and hip anti-gravity extension lag greater than 90 degrees, the line of gravity can no longer be maintained (Fig. 39). Walking ends at this point. In this regard, the patient can tolerate knee extension lag better than extension lag of the hip because with fixed ankle equinus the knee can be locked into stabile extension, whereas the hip cannot. The combined extension lag measurement is, of course, without significance, unless enough equinovarus to decrease lower extremity stability is present.

Surgical Technique

Subcutaneous release of tendon contractures permits early mobilization thus obviating the danger of prolonged inactivity. Twenty-four hour skin preparation is desirable as this precludes the need for a long scrub under anaesthesia in a patient whose respiratory exchange is

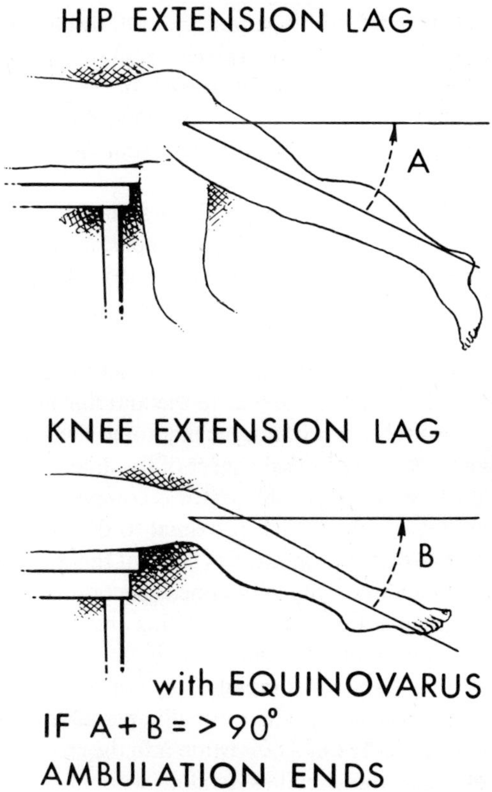

Fig. 39.

usually compromised. A fracture table facilitates postoperative cast application, a double-holed lap sheet completes draping and an adequate array of tenotomes decreases the possibility of infection, assuring that no knife need be used more than once in any wound.

The danger of damage to important neurovascular structures such as the femoral artery in the groin or the common peroneal nerve at the knee, can be avoided by marking these sites with methylene blue.

A word concerning anaesthesia. Suxamethonium should not be used. Some muscular dystrophics are also sensitive to Halothane, an anaesthetic which has caused cardiac toxicity and malignant hyperthermia. This may be related to low potassium storage. Additionally, myotonics have an increased sensitivity to thiopentone. These agents should be administered with caution, if at all, to patients with muscle disease undergoing surgery, however brief. Barbiturates depress respiration, and even standard doses of succinylcholine have deleterious effects. The anaesthesiologist should carefully attend cardiac monitoring, provide adequate ventilation and avoid potassium overload and gastric dilatation.

Subcutaneous tenotomy of hip flexors (including sartorius and straight head of rectus femoris) is accomplished by introducing the tenotome at the anterior-superior iliac spine and sweeping it distally and posteriorly. The knife is kept close to bone, and, if this is done while fully flexing the contralateral hip, flexion contracture can usually be decreased by at least 50%. Remaining contracture exists in the deeper hip flexors (e.g. iliopsoas) as well as in the anterior hip capsule.

Through the same stab wound, the tenotome severs the origin of the tensor fasciae latae at the lateral aspect of the anterior portion of the iliac crest. Bipolar tenotomy of the tensor is completed by subcutaneous release of the iliotibial band just proximal to the lateral aspect of the knee joint. Prognosis for correction is better if this structure is taut and narrow rather than thick and ill defined. Section of the lateral intermuscular septum is assured by completing this incision to the bone. Separation of approximately one inch in the palpable ends of the transected iliotibial band, accompanied by correction of tensor fasciae contracture, is thus accomplished. Finally, percutaneous tenotomy of the heel cord is performed at its insertion into the calcaneus. It is important to tenotomize the Achilles tendon without a tourniquet as a hematoma forms quickly in this area and skin does not fall into the space created by separation of the cut ends of the tendon. Dressings or a cast applied with a tourniquet in use encourages such prolapse and can prevent the localization of the hematoma necessary for healing. The entire percutaneous procedure takes less than five minutes (Fig. 40).

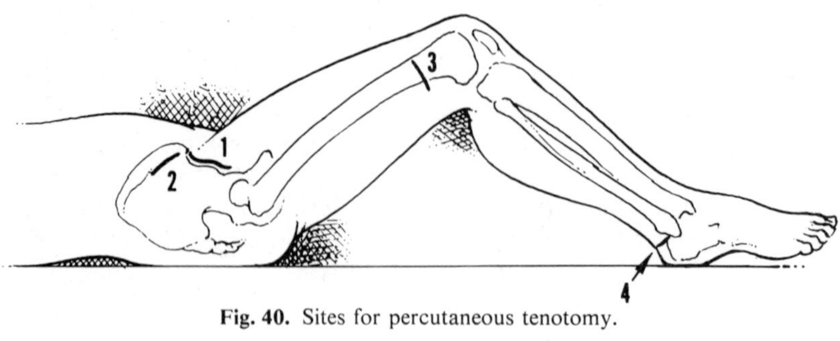

Fig. 40. Sites for percutaneous tenotomy.

If heel cord tenotomies are included in the surgery, toe-to-groin plaster casts are applied with the ankles at neutral and the knees in 5 degrees of flexion. To assure plantigrade position in the casts, the planter surfaces are flattened on a board during application. In those patients in whom heel cord lengthening is not performed (either because it is unnecessary or was done previously), braces are fitted postoperatively.

When casts are applied, they are worn for three weeks, and lower extremity braces are then fitted. These braces feature double uprights, drop-ring locks, spring-loaded ankles with an adjustable stop, sheepskin

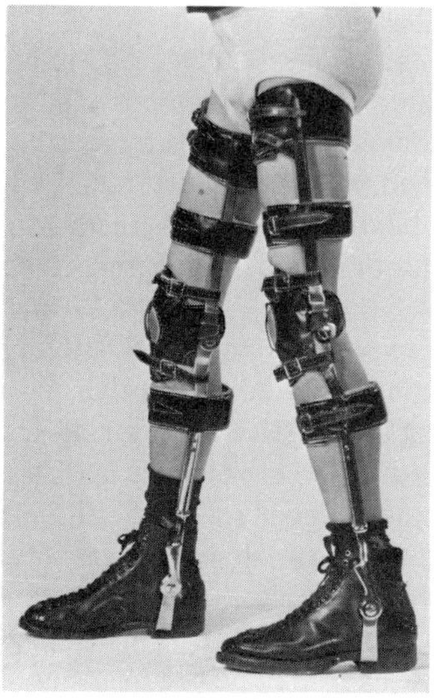

Fig. 41.

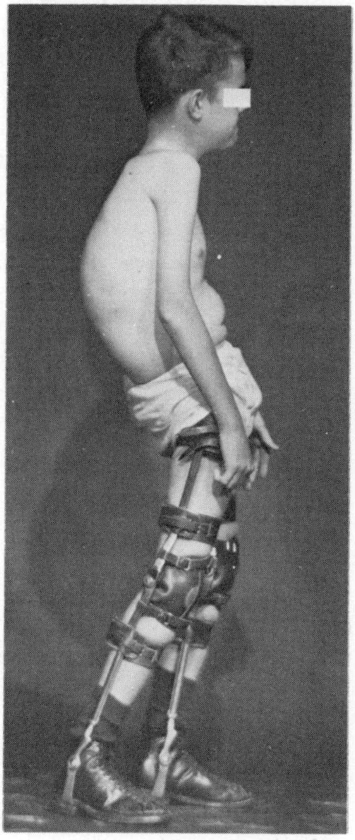

Fig. 42. Kyphosis secondary to short braces.

heel inserts, slight knee flexion, and a contoured proximal leather band which provides further support through ischial seating (Fig. 41). This band must lie just below the ischial tuberosity. If it is too high, the patient will tilt forward out of balance; if too low, a servere kyphosis may develop (Fig. 42). The weight of these braces is approximately 4.5 kg.

With proper attention brace ambulating children seldom fall. More fractures occur from falling from a wheelchair or bed than from falls in braces. As braces require lengthening, care must be taken not to bring the proximal band higher than 2 cm below the ischial tuberosity else the braces will not permit necessary ischial seating and the patient will not be able to walk.

Preoperative knee contractures of more than 20 degrees are corrected in serial casts to 5 degrees or less. Surgical correction of knee contractures has not been found necessary although release of the tensor fasciae incidently corrects some knee contracture as this structure plays a role in knee flexion.

Heel cord lengthening as an isolated procedure will not be successful if the quadriceps is weak unless long-leg bracing accompanies the surgery. However, heel cord lengthening can permit better balance in patients already walking with long-leg braces. On the other hand, section of the iliotibial band can delay bracing and improve walking balance both before and after bracing.

Postoperative care includes the brief use of nasal oxygen and intermittent positive pressure breathing. A Circolectric bed is used, and, on the afternoon of surgery, the patient stands in bed with his feet resting on the footboard attachment. When in bed, he is positioned to stretch the hips into extension and adduction by binding the legs together at the knees and elevating the sacrum when on his back and the knees when on his abdomen.

Because subcutaneous tenotomy minimizes pain and the possibility of wound dehiscence, physical therapy can be started on the afternoon of surgery. Treatment consists of standing and passive hip exercise. On the first postoperative day, the patient is walked. If in casts, the heels are fish-mouthed to avoid pressure, the bottoms pounded soft, and adhesive tape is applied for friction. This is more stable than rubber walkers, and, providing firmer floor contact, reinforces the kinesthetic supporting response.

Initially, the use of a light aluminium walker may be necessary until the patient adjusts to his rediscovered balance. Although he finds that during walking it is still necessary to shift his torso over the supporting limb, the exaggerated postures of head and shoulder extension, as well as the severe lumbar lordosis which were a preoperative necessity for body alignment, are no longer required. Lumbar lordosis disappears when these children sit and they walk sitting on their braces with a penguin (or Alderman's) type gait.

Almost all day is spent in the therapy department, and most of that time the child is standing or walking. This is continued for the better part of a week, when he is discharged to a programme of home physical therapy including passive hip stretching and walking. Casts are discarded three weeks after surgery, and for the next three months, except for removal for skin care, braces are worn day and night. It is most urgent that mobility skills once regained not be soon lost again.

Although tennis shoes are best for patients out of braces because they are light and their rubber soles provide traction, high-laced surgical boots are the footwear of choice for the braced patient. However, a lighweight plastic brace is now available. Because it incorporates a moulded foot-plate, special shoes are unnecessary for its use. Such a brace is ischial weight-bearing and moulded from 5 mm stress relieved semiopaque polypropylene. Any type of standard knee joint can be incorporated in the appliance. Although the final weight of the average brace is 0.68 kg (less than one third of the standard double upright steel and leather appliance, and less than one half of its aluminium counterpart), these orthoses maintain a high strength/weight ratio.

Ankle mobility in the orthosis is regulated by varying the width of the posterior strut connecting the calf piece to the foot plate. The plastic is moulded with the ankle in dorsiflexion and the strut then trimmed until slight plantar flexion and rotation are possible.

Because the upright supporting members of the appliance are form-fitted from plastic, it is less bulky than a standard brace, more comfortable and quite cosmetically acceptable. Either buckle or Velcro fittings can be used for closure and the entire leg piece hidden underneath a long stocking.

Finally, all materials (including the knee pad which can be fabricated from plastizoate and Velcro, and fittings which can be made of aluminum) are nontoxic, radiolucent, unaffected by oils or ultraviolet light and completely waterproof. Thus, the appliance can be washed and dried with ease, a feature contrasting severely with the difficulty of cleaning the leather utilized in the ordinary brace.

Because it is difficult to switch a patient from the standard double upright brace to its plastic counterpart, it is suggested that if the plastic orthosis is to be used at all, it should be the initial brace provided.

Even after wheelchair confinement the stability afforded by braces is appreciated by most patients as the cosmetically acceptable alignment of the lower extremities is maintained.

Because the posterior tibial muscles remain strong despite progression of weakness in other musculature, they have been transferred by Spencer through the interosseous membrane and inserted through a drill hole in the third cuneiform by means of O-chromic suture tied over a bolster on the bottom of the foot. This procedure has strengthened dorsiflexion and eversion of the foot by eliminating the force of the posterior tibial, which may cause a recurrence of equinovarus deformity. The occasional case of isolated forefoot equinus can be treated with midtarsal capsulectomy and percutaneous plantar fasciotomy.

Even in patients confined to bed the tibialis posticus and toe flexors have been graded as fair plus. This transfer, however, does not work in phase but rather on command because the tibialis posticus is a stance phase muscle and, when transferred to the dorsum, becomes a swing phase muscle. However, relocation of its insertion removes an overactive tendency to inversion, providing an active eversion tenodesis effect. This operation is best performed early, as a prophylactic procedure, before severe plantar soft tissue contracture or bony deformity in the foot have occurred.

Muscle tissue comprises 50% of total body weight, and although over half of this muscle mass is lost by the end of independent abulation, by which time patients are sometimes too weak to stand alone, they are often able to walk again after correction of contractures and bracing. This is because other factors are also influential in preventing ambulation. Joint contracture due to disproportionate agonist-antagonist strength, diffuse atrophy because of decreasing physical activity, obesity, emotional problems and wheelchair immobilization imposed for the convenience of others all play a role in limiting walking potential.

Complications of lower extremity surgery may include heel decubitus ulcer, anterolateral thigh numbness (secondary to transsection of anterior branch of the lateral femoral cutaneous nerve), or any of the usual postoperative problems occurring even after short anaesthesia and relatively bloodless surgery in a patient with poor respiratory toilet and generalized weakness. Fortunately, the incidence and degree of these complications have been minimal.

The usual time for surgery and bracing is between nine and twelve years of age.* The patient so treated can handle his toilet needs with minimal help and chair transfer is facilitated by locking his braces at the knees and using the legs as a long lever to tilt the patient to the standing position. The average interval of extended ambulation beyond surgery is from three to five years. This additional period of ambulation may represent up to 20% of the life span of these children and is thus a highly significant benefit to them as maintenance of the upright posture has extended their ability to attend to all the tasks of daily living for a significant portion of their lives.

BIBLIOGRAPHY

Cobham, I. G. and Davis, H. S. (1964), 'Anesthesia for Muscle Dystrophy Patients,' *Anesthesia and Analgesia*, **43,** No. 1, 22–29.

Cohen, P. J. (1972), 'Halogenated Anesthetic and Patients with Elevated CPK Level,' *J. Amer. med. Ass.* (Questions and Answers), **220,** No. 9, 1253.

Eyring, E. J., Johnson, E. W. and Burnett, Carol P. T. (1972), 'Surgery in Muscular Dystrophy,' *J. Amer. med. Ass.*, **222,** No. 8, 1056–1057.

Gucker III, T. (1964), 'The Orthopedic Management of Progressive Muscular Dystrophy,' *J. Amer. Phys. Ther. Ass.*, **44,** No. 4, 243–246.

Isaacs, H. and Barlow, B, (1973), 'Malignant Hyperpyrexia. Further Muscle Studies in Asymptomatic Carriers Identified by Creatinine Phosphokinase Screening,' *J. Neurol. Neurosurg. Psychia.*, **36,** No. 2, 228–243.

Miller, Jo (1967) 'Management of Muscular Dystrophy,' *J. Bone J. Surg.*, **49-A,** No. 6, 1205–1211.

Roy, L. and Gibson, D. A. (1970), 'Pseudohypertrophic Muscular Dystrophy and its Surgical Management: Review of 30 patients,' *Canad. J. Surg.*, **13,** 13–21.

Siegel, I. M. (1975), 'Plastic-Molded Knee-Ankle-Foot Orthoses in the Treatment of Duchenne Muscular Dystrophy,' *Arch. Phys. Med. Rehab.*, **56,** 322.

Siegel, I. M., Miller, J. E. and Ray, R. D. (1968), 'Subcutaneous Lower Limb Tenotomy in the Treatment of Pseudohypertrophic Muscular Dystrophy,' *J. Bone J. Surg.*, **50A,** 1437–1443.

* Almost 50% of patients will stop walking by age 9. Comparison of affected brothers shows that the age at which walking ceased did not differ by more than one year in most cases and by more than 3 years in any instance.

Spencer, G. E., Jr. (1967), 'Orthopaedic Care of Progressive Muscular Dystrophy,' *J. Bone Jt. Surg.*, **49A,** No. 6, 1201–1204.

Spencer, G. E., Jr. and Vignos, J. P., Jr. (1962), 'Bracing for Ambulation in Childhood Progressive Muscular Dystrophy,' *J. Bone Jt. Surg.*, **44A,** No. 2, 234–242.

Spencer, G. E., Jr. (1973), 'Orthopaedic Considerations in the Mangement of Muscular Dystrophy,' in *Recent Advances in Orthopaedics,* Chapter 11, pp. 279–293 (J. Ahstrom, Ed.). Baltimore, Md.: Williams & Wilkins Co.

Vignos, P. J., Jr. and Archibald, K. C. (1960), 'Maintenance of Ambulation in Childhood Muscular Dystrophy,' *J. Chronic Dis.*, **12,** No. 2, 273–290.

Ziter, F. A. and Allsop, K. G. (1975), 'Comprehensive Treatment of Childhood Muscular Dystrophy,' *Rocky Mtn med. J.*, **72,** No. 8, 329–333.

CHAPTER 16

Surgical Treatment: Foot Deformity

Equinocavovarus deformity was noted by Duchenne in his original description of pseudohypertrophic muscular dystrophy (Fig. 43). As the disease progresses and weakness and contracture increase, this deformity jeopardizes alignment stability in the lower extremities, and is by far the most serious foot deformity in the musclar dystrophies. Foot drop secondary to tibialis anticus weakness in facioscapulohumeral dystrophy and the steppage gait due to weak dorsiflexion in dystrophia myotonica can both be managed with light wire spring drop foot bracing or a floor reaction orthoses. If these appliances do not help, a standard double upright ankle brace with a Klenzak spring dorsiflexion assist will usually correct the deformity. Such an appliance may even be necessary in the later stages of limb-girdle dystrophy. However, in classical Duchenne disease a rapidly progressive weakening of foot musculature with contracture occurs and although this may respond temporarily to conservative measures such as passive stretch, surgical correction is ultimately necessary.

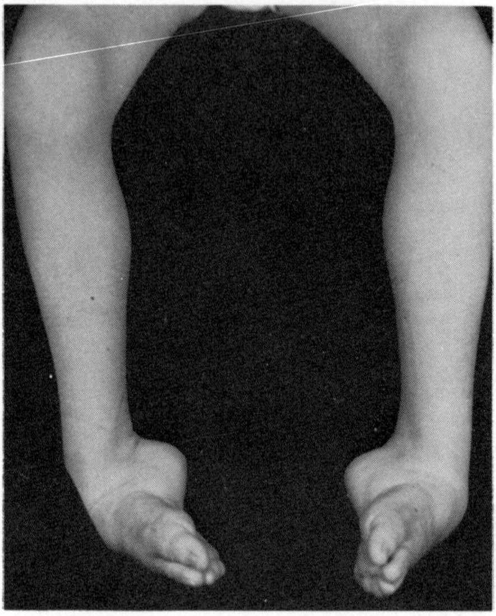

Fig. 43. Equinocavovarus deformity.

Passive Stretching

Overenthusiastic stretching of foot contracture should be avoided. This causes pain which prompts the patient to fight the passive force by an active effort of his own. The stretch reflex is also stimulated and this action results in strengthening of the deforming muscle or muscles. As we have seen, heel cord contracture is usually more severe on one side because of the position of haunch habitually taken. Thus, one foot is held in advance of the other, the partially flexed extremity developing the more severe heel cord contracture.

Equinocavovarus

Equinocavovarus advances because of a selective weakening of foot musculature. The tibialis anticus is weakened early but not the gastrocnemius. Contracture of the heel cord with its eccentric medial calcaneal insertion, augmented by unopposed tibialis posterior and toe flexor tension, forces the foot into this deformity. Rotation at the talocalcaneal joint, whose surfaces lie in an oblique anterolateral position encourages forefoot supination. Once the foot is inverted beyond the tibiotalar sagittal midline, almost all dorsal and volar musculature, intrinsic and extrinsic, works to invert it further (Fig. 44).

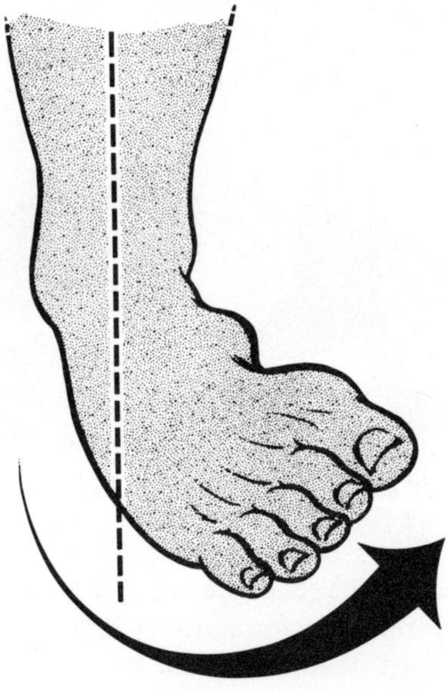

Fig. 44.

Progressive equinocavovarus makes standing and walking uncomfortable and difficult. Pressure decubiti can develop and the deformity will eventually prevent maintenance of the upright posture. Equinocavovarus is particularly disabling when combined with flexion-abduction hip contracture. In spite of correction of the hip deformity, equinocavovarus can continue.

Attempts to forestall this condition, utilizing lateral sole and heel wedging, outer T-straps and corrective shoe inserts* (Fig. 45) may be temporarily successful, but surgical correction is eventually necessary.

Bony deformity precludes the use of soft tissue release alone. Although realignment of the foot can usually be obtained through the

* e.g. the University-of-California–Berkeley (UCB) insert, which determines forefoot supination-pronation by controlling heel valgus-varus.

standard techniques of triple arthrodesis or midtarsal wedge resection, these patients suffer rapid loss of strength when inactive. Operations such as these are contraindicated as they require prolonged postoperative immobilization to assure bone fusion and soft tissue healing without dehiscence of multisutured surgical wounds.

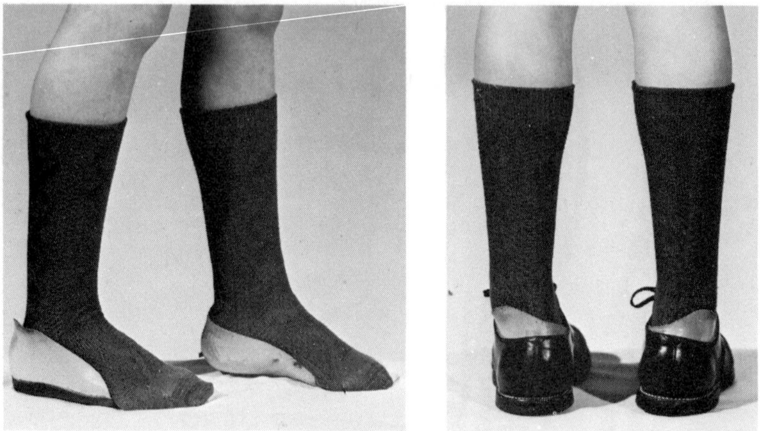

Fig. 45. Plastic corrective shoe inserts.

However, early in the sequence of this deformity when equinus alone is the major deforming factor and very little cavus or varus is present, isolated heel cord tenotomy can be performed. But heel cord lengthening or tenotomy removes the stabilizing force which hyperextends and locks the knee during stance so that nonbraced ambulation is usually impossible unless the quadriceps is better than fair strength.

Later, when all elements of the deformity are present, a more extensive surgical attack is necessary. Percutaneous tarsal medullostomy, combined with soft tissue release and posterior tibial tenotomy, can correct equinocavovarus, enabling the patient to stand the night of surgery and walk the next day.

Technique

A 24-hour surgical skin preparation is used. Under tourniquet control a stab wound is placed over the dorsal aspect of the mid-tarsal area centering on the talar head. A large curette is introduced into the talar head which is then echolated of cancellous bone. The distal calcaneus is similarly treated, when necessary, either through the same or a separate stab wound.

Percutaneous plantar fasciotomy is performed to correct cavus. The tendon of tibialis posticus is identified distal to the medial malleolus and tenotomized percutaneously. Deformity is corrected by manipulation of the foot with collapse of the curetted bones (Fig. 46). If single stitch

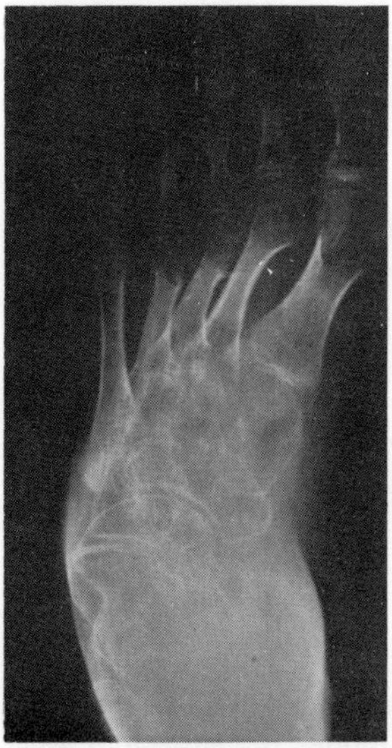

Fig. 46. a.
A.P. view of foot prior to procedure.

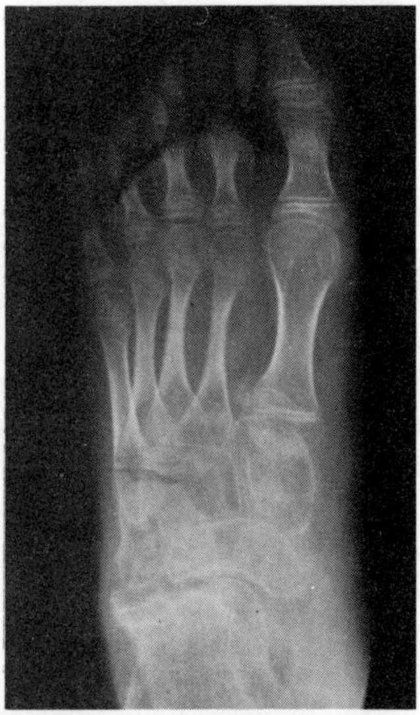

Fig. 46. b.
A.P. view of foot after procedure.

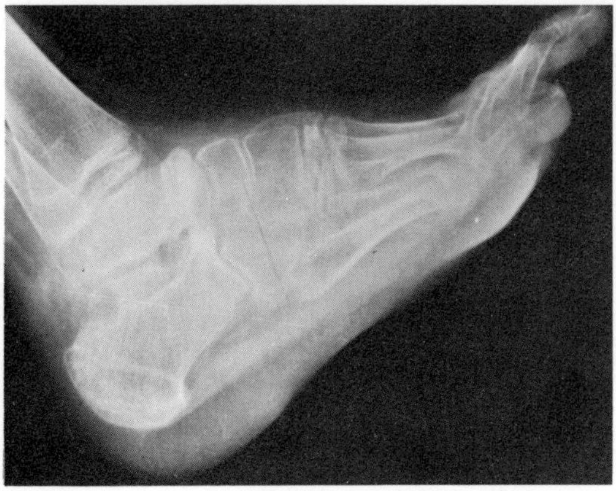

Fig. 46. c.
Lateral view of foot after procedure.

wound closure is necessary, 3–0 plain catgut is used. A well-padded, long leg plaster is applied. The cast is split, its heel portion 'fish-mouthed', and the sole pounded soft.

The patient is encouraged to stand the evening of surgery and ambulate the next day. The use of a walker may be necessary for a brief period until balance is rediscovered. Casts are worn for three weeks, followed by a return to long leg braces.

For wheelchair confined patients, where there is no further need to stand and ambulate, advanced equinocavovarus is treated by the simple expedient of mid-tarsal dorso-lateral closing wedge osteotomy.

Infrequently, forefoot adductus is found as a residual or recurrent deformity. Percutaneous metatarsal osteotomy utilizing a thin osteotome introduced through three dorsal stab wounds can correct this deformity permitting early postoperative ambulation in a corrective cast. In cases with residual weakness from polymyositis, tibialis anticus is sometimes active and can be transferred to the dorso-lateral aspect of the foot thus removing a deforming inversion force and creating an active dorsiflexor in neutral or eversion.

Correction of lower extremity instability is mandatory because even minor degrees of contracture in weight-bearing joints can interfere with balance and reduce the ability to ambulate. Relatively simple surgical procedures are available and a judicious choice among these, followed by almost immediate postoperative ambulation, can prolong walking. As the patient's ability to stand and walk diminish the physician must determine whether this is the result of contracture or weakness. Experience has shown that where indicated the earlier surgery is done the better the ensuing result. All surgery should be bilateral if possible so that symmetrical posture can be maintained. The subcutaneous procedures here described enable patients to maintain and significantly extend the ability to ambulate independently, thus delaying wheelchair or bed confinement.

BIBLIOGRAPHY

Siegel. I. M. (1972), 'Equinocavovarus in Muscular Dystrophy,' *Arch. Surg.*, **104,** 644–646.

CHAPTER 17

Treatment: Scoliosis

Occurrence

Scoliosis in muscular dystrophy appears to occur with increasing age and advancing disability. Its presence depends upon the type of dystrophy present; its progress is related to the severity of the primary disease. Childhood dystrophia myotonica is not complicated by spinal curvature because axial, shoulder and pelvic musculature are weakened only late in this condition. The onset of limb girdle dystrophy is usually in middle or late adolescence. Weakness is most often symmetrical and progression slow. Patients are ambulatory into the second or third decade, deformities occur late, and scoliosis is an uncommon finding. When it does occur, spinal growth has most often terminated and the deformity is functional rather than structural.

In the case of the Duchenne form of dystrophy, there is also symmetrical muscular involvement and weakness, but the patient is usually younger and vertebral growth is still in progress. Structural curvature is initiated by mechanical disequilibrium (increased gravitational stress secondary to spinal-pelvic malalignment) and appears unrelated to paralysis or asymmetry of axial muscle strength.

Where lower extremity contracture is relieved by tenotomy and long leg bracing, pelvic or infrapelvic tilt are obviated as factors in the production of scoliosis. Properly braced patients walk with a stiff-legged gait, modulating the centre of mass over the standing hip joint with each successive step. Because torso shift is necessary for balance, the use of rigid body support would inhibit ambulation and is contraindicated. The oscillation of body weight necessitates alternating lateral spinal bending, providing excellent symmetrical spinal exercise during ambulation, thus inhibiting the production of static spinal curvature.

In those patients with untreated hip, knee and ankle contractures, several factors contribute to early spinal deformity. Most of these children stand in a haunched position, with one foot advanced for balance. This tilts the pelvis, producing a compensatory scoliotic deformity. Asymmetrical arm position can also cause secondary spinal deviation. Body alignment requires use of the upper extremities as stabilizing appendages (much as a tightrope walker uses a long pole for balance). Because weak deltoid muscles cannot maintain shoulder abduction, the patient hooks his thumbs over his brace tops, belt or trouser

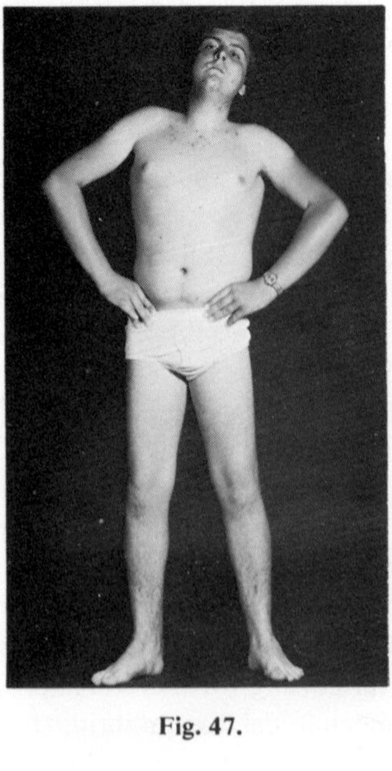

Fig. 47.

pockets, supporting his upper extremities in shoulder extension and internal rotation, elbow flexion and forearm pronation (Fig. 47). This posture is compensatory, necessary for balance and should not be corrected. However, when continued, the arms tend to contract in this position, and any irregularity of upper extremity placement unbalances the torso and bends the spine. When these patients can no longer independently turn in bed, they tend also to develop a dorsal spinal curvature, convex to the side upon which they lie.

Almost all patients which Duchenne dystrophy develop scoliosis rapidly after they can no longer independently stand and walk. This may be delayed by prolonging ambulation as long as possible through early contracture release and bracing. Patients confined to wheelchair after completion of vertebral growth stand a better chance of avoiding lateral structural spinal curvature. Severe rigid lumbar lordosis frequently occurs after prolonged sitting. However this deformity tends to lock the facet joints providing a more mechanically stabile posture than that of kyphosis where these joints are open and more vulnerable to bending and rotational stress.

Bracing

A rigid (celastic or perforated orthoplast isoprene) torso support and a firm level pelvic seat should be provided when wheelchair confinement becomes inevitable, before the onset of spinal curvature (Fig. 48). The patient in a wheelchair supports himself by leaning to the nondominant side while using the dominant arm. He shifts his weight to the nondominant side, tilts his pelvis and produces a spinal curve convex to that direction. These spines are essentially flaccid and respond to the exoskeletal thoraco-pelvic distribution forces such a jacket provides. This frees the arms from a supporting role and encourages spinal soft tissue contracture in a position of acceptable alignment. Spinal alignment is obtained by supporting the abdomen, elevating the ribs from a contoured pelvic foundation* and (utilizing residual neck extension strength) forcing the shoulders back. With correction of abdominal ptosis the diaphragm is allowed increased freedom of movement and vital capacity is thereby enhanced. Such an appliance must be refitted as the child grows. The Milwaukee brace is of little use here as it is a dynamic orthosis, and patients in the later stages of muscle disease lack sufficient strength to exercise in the appliance.

* If the pelvis is stabilized, the critical vertical load necessary to produce lateral spinal deformity must be doubled.

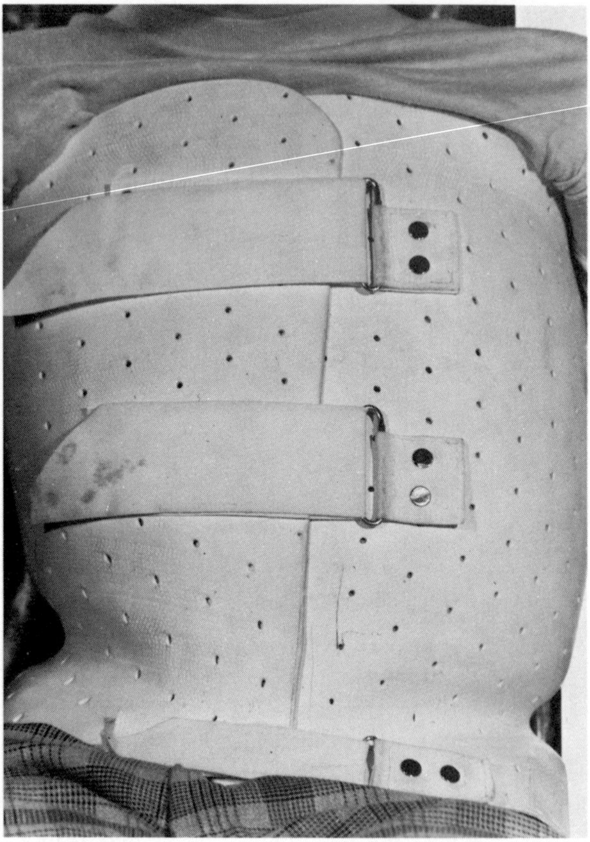

Fig. 48.

Facioscapulohumeral Dystrophy

Facioscapulohumeral dystrophy is rapidly progressive when onset occurs in childhood. It is also one of the few muscular dystrophies which may be asymmetrical in distribution. Thus, scoliosis is not uncommonly seen while patients are still walking, at which time spinal deformity can prevent body alignment and hinder ambulation.

Weakness in this form of dystrophy is usually less than in the other kinds of childhood myopathy, and prognosis for continued function and life expectancy is, as a general rule, more hopeful. These patients tolerate major spinal surgery well, muscle strength permits use of the

Milwaukee brace, and their scolioses are generally amenable to more traditional forms of therapy.

Several illustrative cases follow:

Case 1. A 12-year-old female was first noted to have a left mid-dorsal scoliosis, well compensated at age 10 (Fig. 49). She was treated conservatively with exercise for two-and-a-half years. At that time her curve measured 47 degrees. This was corrected to 10 degrees in a Risser plaster jacket, and her spine fused from D6 to D12 (Fig. 50). She was maintained in plaster for ten months, the first five of which were nonambulatory.

After removal of her cast, she ambulated well, but some weakness of the shoulders was noted. This progressed until definite scapular winging became apparent (Fig. 51). It was now almost three years after spinal fusion. Examination revealed the stigmata of facioscapulohumeral dystrophy, and over the following year weakness and deformity progressed until she developed bilateral foot drop, severe lordosis and the typical facies of this disease (Fig. 52).

At her last examination she was 22 years old, 10 years post-fusion. Her curvature had not progressed and she continued ambulatory. She may have had a typical juvenile idiopathic scoliosis; however, one cannot help but wonder whether immobilization hastened the onset and progress of her primary muscle disease.

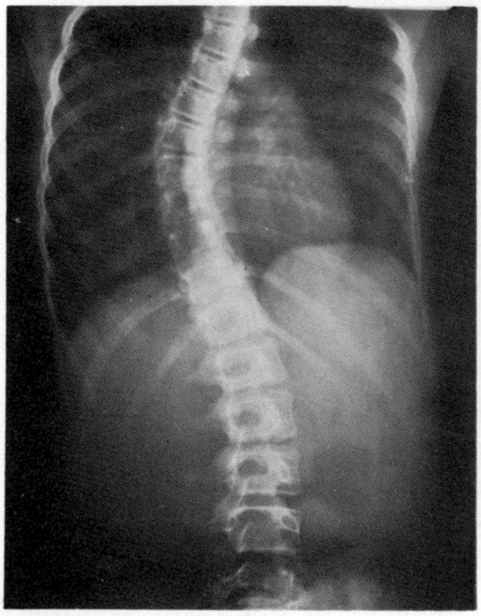

Fig. 49.

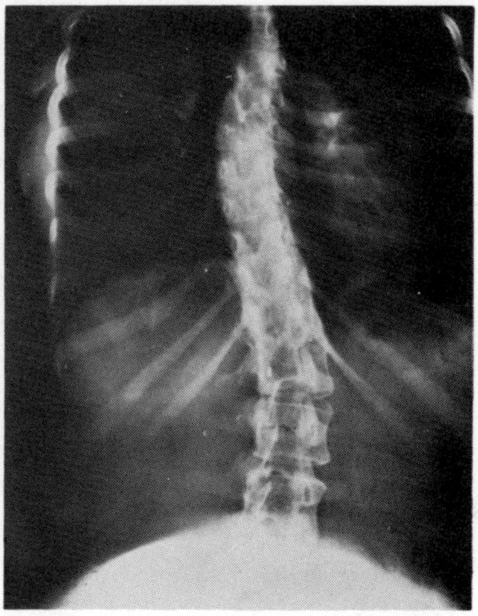

Fig. 50.

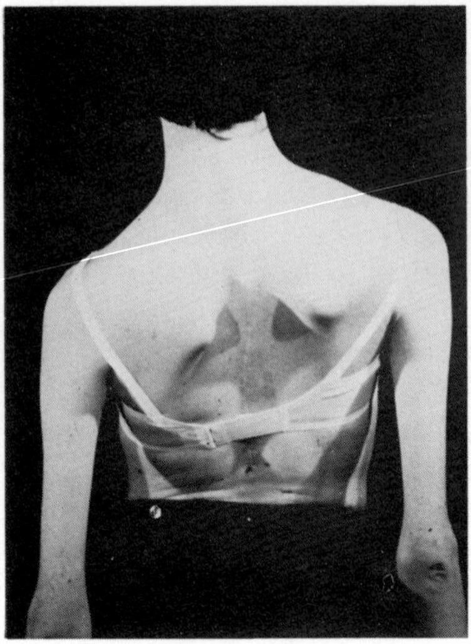

Fig. 51. Scapular winging.

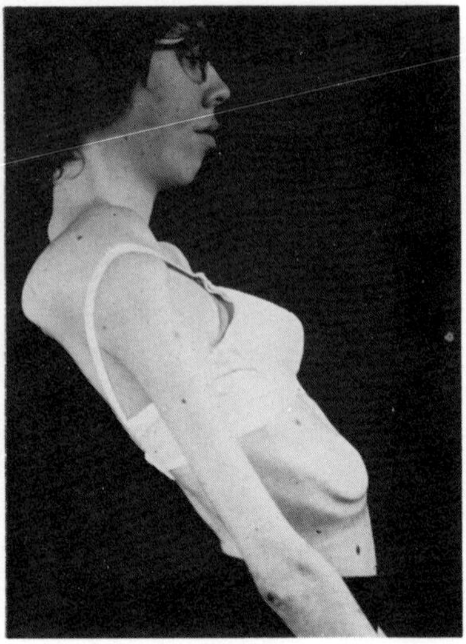

Fig. 52. Facies of facioscapulohumeral dystrophy.

Case 2. A 13-year-old male presented with a far advanced facioscapulohumeral dystrophy. A left cervical, severe long thoracolumbar scoliosis to the right, with marked posterior rib angulation was present (Fig. 53). A Risser type corrective body jacket cast was applied. This improved the patient's gait. His curve was quite flexible in the upper portion and decreased significantly with traction. A localizer cast was fitted and a spinal fusion with Harrington rod instrumentation from D3 to L3 performed (Fig. 54). Shortly after surgery he was allowed up on a tilt table, from where he progressed to parallel bars and a walker. One month later, a halo was applied under local anaesthesia, and this was subsequently attached to a Milwaukee brace. He was ambulated in the halo and brace (Fig. 55). After five months the halo was removed and a standard Milwaukee brace chin piece substituted (Fig. 56).

In spite of a severe collapsing paralytic scoliosis, secondary to far advanced myopathy, this patient tolerated surgery well, and the use of Harrington spinal instrumentation, augmented by the halo and Milwaukee brace, permitted correction of his curve with early mobilization.

In summary, the treatment of scoliosis in muscular dystrophy depends upon the type and degree of myopathy present. Childhood

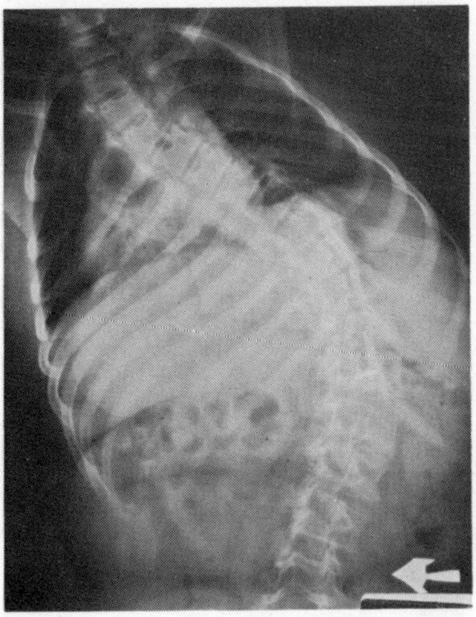

Fig. 53.

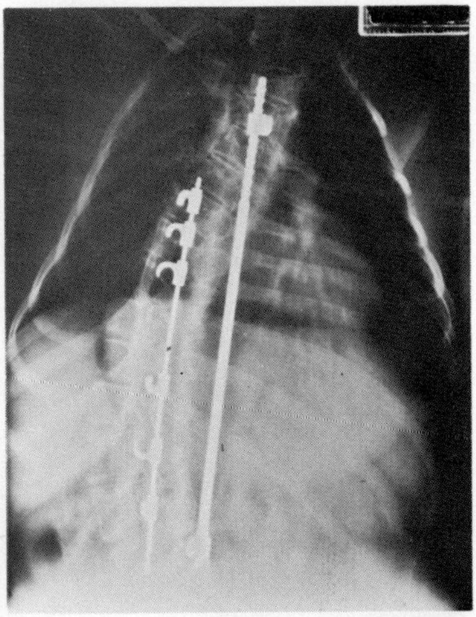

Fig. 54.

myotonia is uncomplicated by spinal curvature. Patients with limb girdle dystrophy, whose onset is usually in middle or late adolescence, and where progress is slow, are often ambulatory well into the third decade and seldom show scoliosis severe enough to warrant treatment.

Duchenne dystrophics develop scoliosis only late during their ambulatory phase* and this can often be avoided by lower extremity contracture release and long leg bracing. Almost all these patients become scoliotic when they can no longer walk. This incidentally has also been noted in spastics (39% of bedridden spastics are scoliotic versus 7% of spastics still ambulatory). As patients with Duchenne dystrophy do not tolerate major spinal operations well†, they are best treated by rigid torso bracing, applied after wheelchair confinement, preferably as prophylactic therapy before the appearance of spinal curvature. The appliance must be fitted early as such patients tend to slump in the wheelchair because it takes less effort than sitting upright and for a time at least, it is more comfortable using the arms from the slumped position.

Currently, the use of internal metallic correction, augmented by methyl methacrylate cement fixation, is being investigated as a means of reducing spinal curvature with minimal surgery. This technique may find application in the Duchenne scoliotic.

* Weakness in 'Becker' dystrophy may be assymetrical and scoliosis can occur while patients are still ambulatory.

† In carefully selected cases, successful spinal fusion has recently been reported.

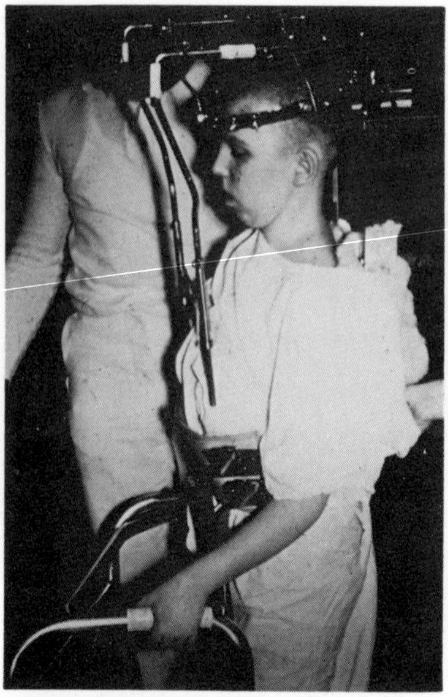

Fig. 55. Ambulation and Halo attached to Milwaukee brace.

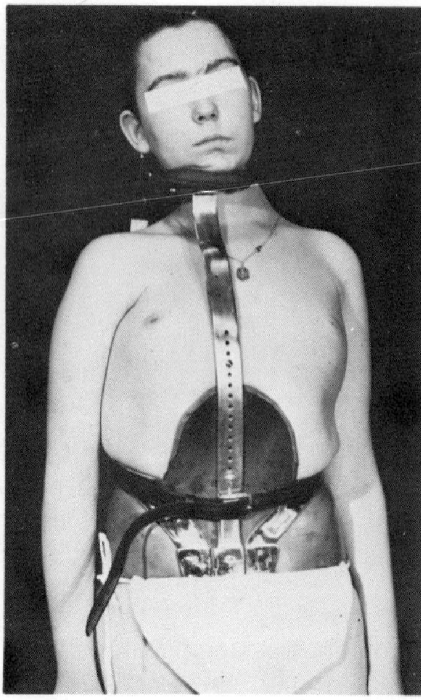

Fig. 56a.

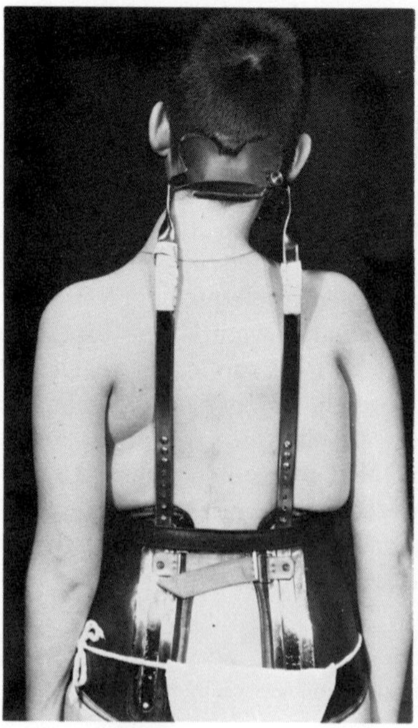

Fig. 56b.

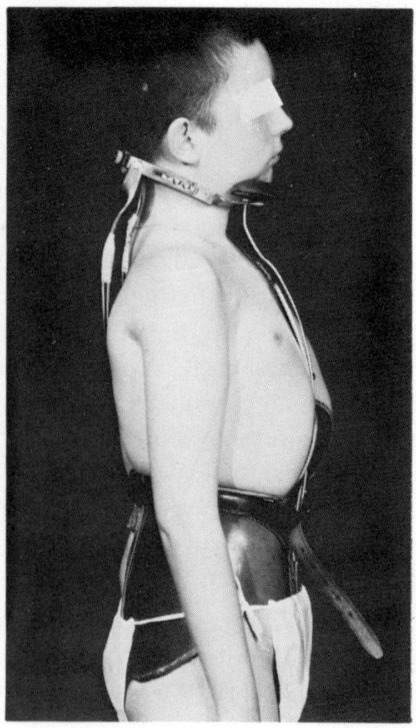

Fig. 56c.

Because facioscapulohumeral dystrophy may be asymmetrical in distribution, structural scoliosis is often a complication of its childhood form and can interfere with balance and walking. However, such patients are amenable to more traditional forms of treatment due to their slow progression and relative maintenance of strength. In selected cases an aggressive programme of surgery and bracing can arrest spinal deformity, thus maintaining ambulatory function.

Finally, some patients with scoliosis, secondary to infantile spinal muscular atrophy and its benign variants are also candidates for spinal fusion and bracing. Generally in these cases, as in muscular dystrophy, the later the onset the less severe the paralysis. The indications for operative intervention in these patients is when the curve is progressive and greater than 30 to 40 degrees in spite of bracing, assuming the course of the neurological disease has stabilized. Such patients require close attention to pulmonary function before, during and after surgery. Because they have a poor pulmonary reserve, surgery will cause an absolute loss of vital capacity for several weeks after operation. This is related to pain, overstretching of intercostal muscles on the convex side of the curve, with relaxation of intercostals on the concave side, compression of the concave lung with over-expansion of the convex lung and decreased reserve in the accessory muscles of respiration.

The prolonged work of postoperative breathing is exhausting to these patients and although they can be managed with an indwelling transnasal or transtracheotomy intertracheal tube, the use of a tank respirator is better tolerated.

BIBLIOGRAPHY

Dunn, H. K. (1972), 'Surgery in the Paralytic Spine.' Personal Communication.

Edelstein, G. (1959), 'Correlation of Handedness and Degree of Joint Contracture in Bilateral Muscle and Joint Disease,' *Amer. J. Phys. Med.*, **38,** 45–47.

Gibson, D. A. and Wilkins, Kay E. (1975), 'The Management of Spinal Deformities in Duchenne Muscular Dystrophy. A New Concept of Spinal Bracing,' *Clinical Orthopaedics and Related Research,* No. 108, pp. 41–51.

Hardy, J. H. (Ed.) (1974), 'Spinal Deformity in Neurological and Muscular Disorders,' 1st Edn., St. Louis: C. V. Mosby Co.

Robin, G. C., Stein, H., Simein, A. and Siegel, I. (1974, 'The Effect of Methacrylate Cement on Loading of Harrington Instruments in the Spine—A Preliminary Experimental Study,' in *Medical and Biological Engineering*, **12,** 241–245.

Siegel, I. M. (1973), 'Scoliosis in Muscular Dystrophy,' in *Clinical Orthopaedics and Related Research*, No. 93, pp. 235–238.

CHAPTER 18

Treatment: Upper Extremities

Intrinsic Hand Muscles

Except in the primary distal myopathies, which are rare, weakness of intrinsic hand musculature is not a serious problem until late in the course of muscular dystrophy. Because of this, patients should be early encouraged in maximal use of the hands for small motor tasks. Even late in the disease, when there is difficulty with self-feeding because hands cannot be raised to the mouth level, ball-bearing aids (see section on wheelchair) can be helpful. Myotonics may have some difficulty in grip release, but this can usually be controlled with medication.

Contractures about the wrist occur most often in flexion. In fact, one of the earliest signs of facioscapulohumeral dystrophy can be a loss of extensor power to a single digit or a weakness of wrist extension. This extension weakness about the hand and wrist occurs later in limb-girdle and progressive muscular dystrophy (Fig. 57).

Elbow flexion contracture with the forearm in pronation is sometimes seen in ambulatory patients with advanced myopathy and eventually seen in all wheelchair confined Duchenne dystrophics where it is accompanied by wrist flexion and ulnar deviation. This position is the one in which the elbow is held most of the time for functional activity. Elbow flexion contracture of up to 15 degrees may even assist the patient in the initiation of further flexion. Severe progression of contracture can be retarded but not prevented by appropriate passive stretching exercises.

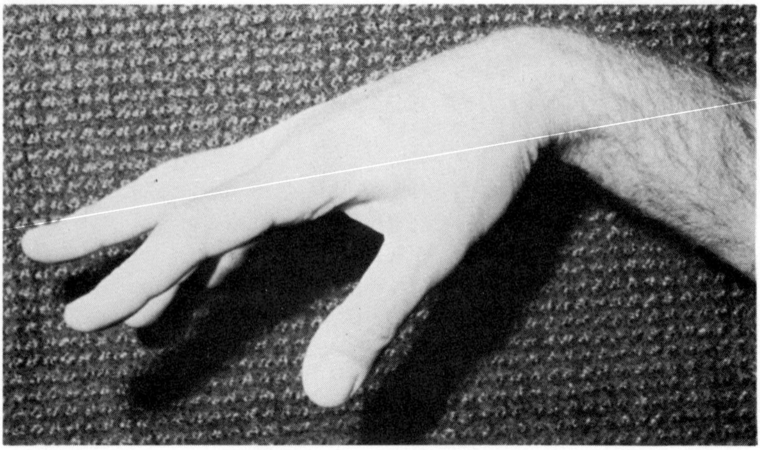

Fig. 57. Lack of finger extension.

Shoulder Contracture

Shoulder contractures in ambulatory Duchenne dystrophics occur because such patients find it necessary to flex the elbow, hooking the thumbs over the side pockets of slacks or through a belt loop, internally rotating the shoulder and pronating the wrist. The elbows are held away from the body and in this way assist in centring the heavy trunk (70% of the body weight) over the pelvis. Internal rotation contracture (but seldom abduction contracture) of the shoulders may be noted. As was mentioned in the chapter on scoliosis, this position is necessary for standing and walking balance and should not be discouraged.

One of the earliest losses in Duchenne dystrophy is that of shoulder stabilization. Serratus anterior can undergo true hypertrophy followed by pseudohypertrophy. Shoulder weakness, manifested by winged scapulae and 'slipping through' is a common finding in early Duchenne and in late limb girdle dystrophy. This represents a weakness of shoulder stabilization (extensors). Deltoid is also frequently involved in the hypertrophic-pseudohypertrophic process (Fig. 58).

It is usually unnecessary to treat shoulder weakness and instability in Duchenne or limb girdle dystrophy. In the Duchenne dystrophic it does not become severe enough to interfere with function until the patient is wheelchair confined at which time it can be treated with assistive appliances. In facioscapulohumeral dystrophy, however, shoulder weakness early significantly interferes with upper extremity function and scapular stabilization should be considered (Fig. 59).

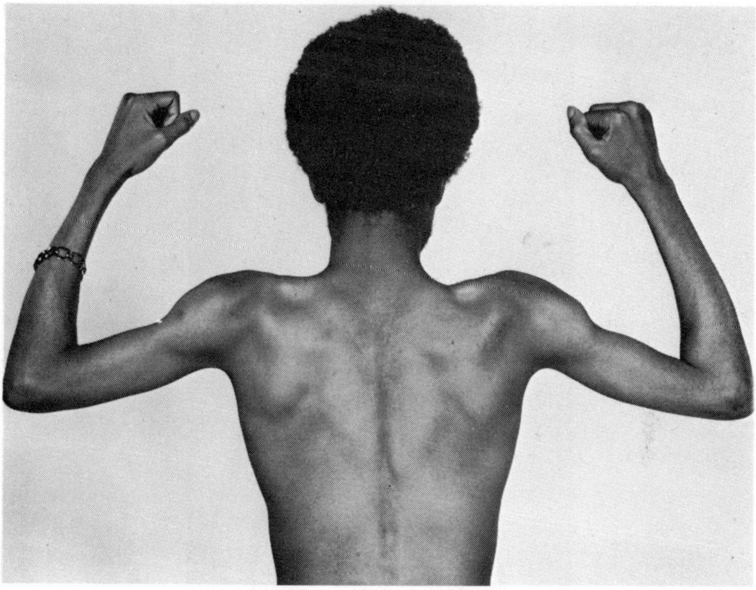

Fig. 58. Deltoid hypertrophy.

These patients find increased difficulty with overhead dressing and, while still ambulatory, cannot bring their hands to their mouths to feed themselves. They find it necessary to flex their necks severely in order to eat. In addition, weakness of scapular adduction aggravates the problem of stance because the shoulders are held anterior to the centre of gravity. This causes an increase of lumbar lordosis and a gait somewhat similar to that seen in Duchenne muscular dystrophy. Because of lack of scapular stability, the deltoids cannot be adequately used, particularly in forward flexion of the arms.

To keep the patient ambulatory, contractures must be stretched and obesity avoided. Special bracing can, at times, help decrease winging of the scapula, lessen scapular adduction, and increase shoulder stability. Braces designed to accomplish this are applied 'figure-of-eight-fashion' around both shoulders, and pads are incorporated to force the scapulae to the chest wall. In selected cases, several surgical procedures are available for scapular stabilization. These include:

1. Interscapular fascial transplant.
2. Screw fixation of scapula to the posterior ribs.
3. Scapular fixation to the posterior ribs through fascial ties.

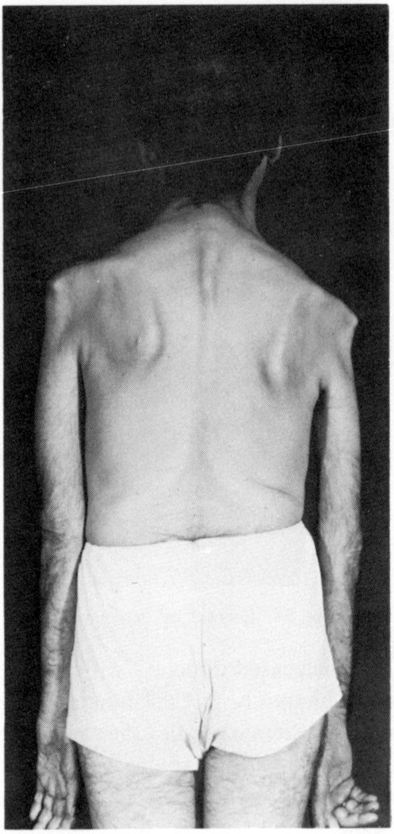

Fig. 59. Shoulder atrophy in facioscapulohumeral dystrophy.

4. Fusion through bone graft between posterior ribs and deep scapular surface, augmented by wire loop fixation of scapula to ribs.

Scapular fixation usually results in about a 10% loss of vital capacity. After scapular stabilization, patients no longer require a 'thrown' movement to elevate the arm. Even slight improvement in abduction is useful when a stabilized scapula provides a firm base for this motion.

Where indicated, it is important to stabilize both the trunk and upper extremities for continued ambulatory balance and sitting stability. In attempting to do this, however, one must take care not to interfere with the physiological compensatory mechanisms of balance which the patient has initiated in an effort to keep himself upright.

BIBLIOGRAPHY

Bunch, W. H. (1973), 'Scapulo-Thoracic Fusion for Shoulder Stabilization in Muscular Dystrophy,' *Minn. Med.*, **56,** 391–394.

Siegel, I. M. (1972), 'Early Signs of Landouzy-Dejerine Disease: Wrist and Finger Weakness,' *J. Amer. med. Ass.*, **221,** No. 3, 302.

Siegel, I. M. (1973), 'Scoliosis in Muscular Dystrophy. Some Comments about Diagnosis, Observations on Prognosis, and Suggestions for Therapy,' in *Clinical Orthopaedics*, No. 93, pp. 235–238.

Walton, J. N. (Ed.) (1974), *Disorders of Voluntary Muscles*, 3rd edition. London: J. & A. Churchill Ltd.

CHAPTER 19

Wheelchair Care

Complications

When all attempts to maintain independent ambulation fail, wheelchair confinement becomes necessary. Although this does not necessarily mark the 'beginning of the end', many complications specific to the use of a wheelchair may require management. These include:

1. Scoliosis.
2. Obesity.
3. Acceleration of cardio-pulmonary difficulties.
4. Decrease in the general rate of all metabolic processes.
5. Reduction of circulation to the lower extremities with dependent edema.
6. Increase of diffuse muscular atrophy, weakness and contracture.
7. Sometimes mental and emotional problems secondary to confinement and almost complete lack of mobility.
8. Functional problems of transfer, feeding, recreation, etc., both for the patient and his family.

Noteworthy is the fact that although such patients sit for most of the day with only an occasional shift of position, pressure decubiti are seldom, if ever, found. Skin subjected to brace or chair pressure, when irritated, can be 'cured' by applying a moist teabag to the area once or twice a day, allowing the liquid to dry on the skin. The mild tannic acid present in the tea toughens the irritated site.

Care

Adequate trunk support must be provided either through padded trunk stabilizers, attached to the wheelchair, or a fitted torso jacket (this was discussed in detail in the section on scoliosis). Trunk supports are not only of value in limiting scoliosis, but position the patient better in his chair, enabling him to use this appliance more effectively. A wide safety belt is always provided.

Although the spine is usually not lordotic while sitting, a firm seat and back (folding inserts providing this are available in various sizes) are desirable for support. In wheelchair-confined adult dystrophics, severe painful lordosis with marked increase in the lumbosacral angle sometimes occurs. This may require corseting for relief. Where neck extension is weak and head control a problem, an extended back rest to support the head becomes necessary.

A wheelchair of appropriate size for each patient is prescribed. This should incorporate large rear wheels, hand brakes, swinging adjustable foot rests with heel straps, an extended head rest, and upholstered, removable desk-type arms (to provide easier transfer to and from toilet and bed). Eight-inch front casters are desirable, and a zipper back for obese patients (permitting them to be placed in a supine position for part of the day to stretch out hip contractures, or for a necessary period of rest) is helpful. Because the narrow doorway to the average bathroom does not permit passage of the standard wheelchair, a combination wheelchair-commode can eliminate the problem of difficult transfer from wheelchair to toilet. Families with limited space seem to prefer this combination to a separate commode.

A portable hydraulic, electric, or mechanical lift facilitates care of those patients who cannot transfer from chair to toilet or bed. One problem with such equipment is its size. In the last phases of wheelchair confinement, an electrically propelled chair may be necessary.

As shoulder function regresses and trunk stability decreases, patients have increased difficulty stabilizing the proximal joints and securing an adequate work area for their hands. Because involvement of distal muscles usually occurs late, it is important that maximal use of the hands be preserved. Lap boards and overhead or ball bearing feeders, which alleviate the gravity load on shoulder and elbow musculature by allowing these weakened muscles to operate across, rather than against, the gravity field, are useful. However, in prescribing aids such as the balanced forearm orthosis, one must consider not only whether the appliance will help the patient, but whether or not the patient will accept the orthosis. Many patients prefer to use even minimal extremity muscle strength, by supporting the elbows on a table and bringing the face to the hands, rather than relying on ball bearing feeders.

In spite of wheelchair confinement, contractures, particularly in the lower extremities, should continue to be stretched. If they are not, non-reducible flexion contracture of the knee and hip can rapidly occur. Daily passive stretch to hips, knees and ankles will prevent acceleration of disabling flexion contracture. Wedges for the feet, holding the ankles in neutral or dorsiflexion, sometimes aid in preventing equinus. Extended leg rests can be used to prevent flexion contracture of the knees.

If the lower extremities are kept supple through stretching, long leg braces can be applied, locked at the knees and ankles, and the patient easily tilted out of his wheelchair by pulling on the belt and/or pushing on his buttocks. This is a considerably easier task than lifting the 'dead weight' of an essentially flail, obese adolescent. Flexibility of soft tissues, especially the two joint muscles in the legs, is particularly important to proper management at this stage of the disease. Once up, considerable psychological and physiological value is obtained through maintenance of an erect posture for at least several hours by using a tilt or standing table. This activity assists in reducing the frequency of static urinary complications and minimizing the degree of diffuse osteoporosis. Another advantage of long leg braces is that they 'set' the patient in his wheelchair, adding weight to the lower portion of his body, thus helping to maintain sitting balance by delaying pelvic tilt.

Obesity should be avoided and a well balanced vitamin-supplemented diet of no less than 1200 calories provided. In the rare case where under-nutrition is a problem, daily food intake can be supplemented with dietary additives containing low potassium hyperalimentatic middle chain triglycerides.

Indeed, wheelchair confinement need not necessarily signal the start of an inexorable downhill course. Although care at this stage is truly 'supportive', maintenance of maximal residual motor power is important to both the patient's functional and emotional well-being.

Chart 11. Occupational Therapy

Name: ____________________

Age: ________

Diagnosis: ____________________

Hand Dominance: ____________________

	Right				*Left*			
Type of Prehension:	*Date*	*Date*	*Date*	*Date*	*Date*	*Date*	*Date*	*Date*
Gross Grasp								
Translation								
Lateral Pinch								
Tip Pinch								
3 Jaw Chuck								
Prehension with:	*Date*	*Date*	*Date*	*Date*	*Date*	*Date*	*Date*	*Date*
Wrist Extended								
Wrist Flexed								

Name: ____________________

Address ____________________ Date: ________

Name: ____________________

Address: ____________________ Date: ________

Name: ____________________

Address: ____________________ Date: ________

Name: ____________________

Address: ____________________ Date: ________

Date: ____________ Birthdate: ____________

Diagnosis: ____________ Appliance: ____________

Therapist: ____________________

Code:
- G: Able to perform activity independently
- Y: Able to perform with one assist, adaptive device, partial performance, too much time
- R: Cannot do
- NA: Not applicable
- NT: Not tested

Classification	*Age**	*Inventory List*	*Date*	*Remarks*	*Date*	*Remarks*	*Date*	*Remarks*
Wheelchair	4	Forward 20 feet						
	4	Backward 5 feet						
	5	Lock, unlock brakes						
	5	Ft. rests and flaps						
Transfers	3	To bed						
	3	From bed						
	3	To chair (st. or arm)						
	3	From chair						
	4	To toilet						
	4	From toilet						
	6	To tub						
	6	From tub						
	3½	Manipulate clothing (Toil)						
	3	Wipe self						
Personal Hygiene	3½	Wash upper extremities						
	3½	Wash lower extremities						
	4	Brush teeth						
	5	Comb hair						
		Shave/Makeup						
	4	Open jars, tubes, etc.						
	3	Turn faucets on and off						
Dressing	3	Shoes on						
	2	Shoes off						
	5	Tie shoes						
	2½	Socks on						
	2	Socks off						
	3	Unbutton shirt						
	4½	Button shirt						
	4	Put shirt on						
	2½	Take shirt off						
	4	Pullover on						
	2½	Pullover off						
	3	Pants on						
	2	Pants off						
	4	Fasten pants						
	3	Unfasten pants						
	4½	Buckle belt						
	3½	Hat on and off						
	2½	Mittens/Gloves						
	4½	Coat on and off						
		Brace, prosthesis, splint						

* Age at which task is normally performed.

Classification	*Age**	*Inventory List*	*Date*	*Remarks*	*Date*	*Remarks*	*Date*	*Remarks*
Feeding	2	Drink from cup (full)						
	3	Drink from glass (full)						
	2½	Drink from straw						
	3	Utensil feed						
	6	Cut with a knife						
		Special feeding device						
Miscellaneous		Glasses on and off						
		Pick up items from floor						
		Telephone						
		Write name and address						

History:

Schooling:
Avocation and Sports Interests:
Adaptive Equipment:

Handedness:
Name and Address: ______________________________
____

Additional Comments:

Occupational Therapy (OT) can play an important role in assessing and assisting the patient at this phase of his disease, and an occupational therapist should be consulted for this purpose. A standard OT evaluation is outlined in Chart 11.

BIBLIOGRAPHY

'Around the Clock Aids for the Child with Muscular Dystrophy.' Muscular Dystrophy Association of America, Inc. Pub. No. P146.

Cherry, Dianne B. (1973), 'Transfer Techniques for Children with Muscular Dystrophy,' *Phys. Ther.*, **53,** No. 9, 970–971.

Chyatte, S. B., Long II, C. and Vignos, P. J., Jr. (1965), 'The Balanced Forearm Orthosis in Muscular Dystrophy,' *Arch. phys. Med. Rehab.*, **46,** 633–636.

McKenzie, Mary W. and Rogers, J. E. (1973), 'Use of Trunk Supports for Severely Paralyzed People,' *Amer. J. Occup. Ther.*, **27,** No. 3, 147–148.

Morris, Ann G. and Vignos, P. J., Jr. (1960), 'A Self-care Program for the Child with Progressive Muscular Dystrophy,' *Amer. J. Occup. Ther.*, **XIV,** No. 6, 301–305.

Summary

Muscular dystrophy is the general designation for a group of chronic diseases whose most prominent characteristic is the progressive degeneration of skeletal musculature.

Although any of the voluntary muscles can be affected, axial musculature and that of the limb girdles is most frequently and most profoundly involved. These diseases are, for the most part, hereditary conditions although spontaneous occurrence, as a result of genetic neomutation is not uncommon. The genetic pattern and, therefore, the mechanism by which the disease is transmitted varies in the different types of dystrophy.

As a rule, it can be said that the earlier clinical symptoms appear, the more rapid is the progression of the disease. The primary pathology, in all types of dystrophy, appears to lie in the muscle cell itself. However, the nervous system may be indirectly or (as recent work has suggested), directly involved in the basic lesion.

No treatment has as yet been found to correct the underlying pathology nor to arrest the relentless progression of muscular dystrophy. Nonetheless, a knowledge of these diseases and their differential diagnosis is important for purposes of treatment, prognosis, detection of carriers in the sex-linked variety and genetic counselling. Accurate diagnosis is vital in the case of inflammatory myopathy where a specific treatment is available. A diagnosis need not entirely depend upon history and clinical examination alone. Electrodiagnosis is available as well as serum muscle enzyme quantification and muscle biopsy.

Once diagnosis is established, management should be prospective consisting of supportive and symptomatic therapy with particular attention paid to cardiomyopathy, pulmonary complications, psychological and social problems. Progressive disability can be delayed by a variety of physiatric and orthopaedic techniques. Serial functional assessment aids in determining the functional stage of the disease and indicating specific therapies. Occupational therapy is utilized to assist the patient in meeting the needs of his activities of daily living within the restrictions imposed by his disease. Physical therapy aids in augmenting strength and relieving contractures through passive stretch. Orthopaedics provides techniques for the surgical relief of lower extremity contractures, the correction of foot and ankle deformity, in selected cases the correction of scoliosis, stabilization of the shoulder, etc. Progressive disability can be delayed by a variety of physiatric techniques including appropriate orthoses and bracing. After patients are no longer ambulatory they require wheelchairs and a variety of special devices to facilitate ongoing care.

Proper treatment of the patient with muscle disease is multidisciplined and aggressive—thus can we minimize the frustrating aspects of these conditions while maximizing the benefits obtained through available care, ever striving to enhance the quality of life.

Index